JUMPING
FOR
HEALTH

A GUIDE TO REBOUNDING AEROBICS

JUMPING

FOR

HEALTH

A GUIDE TO REBOUNDING AEROBICS

Morton Walker, D.P.M.

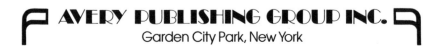
AVERY PUBLISHING GROUP INC.
Garden City Park, New York

The medical and health procedures in this book are based on the training, personal experiences, and research of the author. Because each person and situation is unique, the publisher urges the reader to check with a qualified health professional before using any procedure where there is any question as to its appropriateness.

The publisher does not advocate the use of any particular diet and exercise program, but believes that the information presented in this book should be available to the public. If you have a history of back troubles, or other physical restrictions, we recommend that you consult with your health care provider before beginning any exercise program.

Because there is always some risk involved, the author and publisher are not responsible for any adverse effects or consequences resulting from the use of any of the suggestions, preparations, or procedures in this book. Please do not use the book if you are unwilling to assume the risk. Feel free to contact a physician or other qualified health professional. It is a sign of wisdom, not cowardice, to seek a second or third opinion.

Cover Design by: Rudy Shur and Marty Hochberg
Cover Photograph by: Tommy Muller
In-House Editor: Nancy Marks Papritz

Library of Congress Cataloging in Publication Data
Walker, Morton.
   Jumping for health : a guide to rebounding aerobics / Morton Walker.
      p.   cm.
   Rev. ed. of: Rebounding aerobics / by Morton Walker and Frank A. Angelo. c1981.
   Includes index.
   ISBN 0-89529-413-3 : $9.95
      1. Trampolining. 2. Trampolining–Physiological aspects.
I. Walker, Morton. Rebounding aerobics. II. Title.
RA781.15.W34   1989
613.7'1–dc19   89-265
                                                     CIP

Printed in the United States of America

10 9 8 7 6

Contents

To Pauline and Arthur Ladds, my friends

Preface

This book offers information for your extraordinary physiological benefit. If you want to live longer having the highest level of wellness and the finest quality of life, continue reading to the end. You'll learn about rebounding and how to gain its prodigious aerobic effects for your own body.

Jumping for Health describes a cellular exercise, not just movement of the human skeleton with its various muscular attachments. Rebounding is different from other activities in labor, recreation, and sports, because it puts gravity to work in your favor. By subjecting each of the 60 trillion cells in your body to greater gravitation pull (G force), waste products are squeezed out and nutrition drawn in. The cells grow healthier and function more efficiently. Regular exposure to this exercise places your entire metabolism at the healthiest plateau of activity.

Furthermore, cell walls grow stronger from each cell demanding more protein from the body. The thicker protein-packed walls hold off foreign invaders, toxins, poisons, and other pollutants more effectively. They keep the cellular protoplasm protected and functioning optimally. Everything improves: the blood, the brain, the lungs, all the internal organs, those of the senses, the muscles, and more. You feel an overall sense of greater well-being.

Rebounding offers the ultimate in exercise, and what we have written here explains almost everything currently known about it. Still, new discoveries are being announced repeatedly, so that more knowledge on the activity will likely be added in the near future.

The author and the publisher anticipate this book will become one of a series of informational texts developing the study of *reboundology. This alternative exercise science has the potential for claiming a place among the main holistic methods in the prevention and treatment of degenerative disease. But right now, your use of this book will immediately help you to increase your span of vision, improve your educational capabilities, stabilize your balance and coordination, rid yourself of addictions, slow down the aging process, reduce the incidence of stress from your life, and do numerous other good things, not the least of which is to keep away heart attack and cancer.

Thus, even while more benefits remain to be documented, many are detailed with these pages. *Reboundology, building on the information foundation in *Jumping for Health* has skyscraper dimensions to which it will rise. This new exercise science is merely in its infancy. There is much to be gained for regular daily rebounding.

For example, by bouncing up and down on the rebound unit your heart becomes stronger even without increasing its heart rate. Why? Because as you come down on the rebounding device you put greater gravitational force on the heart muscle. Any muscle automatically adjusts to its environment; in this case, the heart muscle fibers grow in strength. Not only that, all of the muscle layers within arterial walls grow stronger, too.

Another example: Since the veins and lymphatic vessels contain one-way valves comprising a hydraulic pressure system, any up-and-down motion repeatedly opens and closes these valves. A natural pumping action ensues. Enhancement of the entire blood circulation and the waste removal system in the body takes place. As a fringe benefit, the cause of varicose veins is eliminated; they tend to fade away.

---

*Reboundology is the study of the effects of the combination of rebound exercise, proper nutrition, and proper mental attitude on the human body. Copyright 1980, National Institute of Reboundology and Health Inc., Edmonds, WA 98020.

In brief, rebounding aerobics is nothing more than a physiological change within the body that promotes a healthier condition from an inferior state of wellness. This change is the body's way of adapting to its new improved condition, achieved through increased activity and assisted by gravity. Adaptation includes various signs of good health such as greater muscular strength, endurance, flexibility, and a reduction in the resting heart rate, blood pressure, and body fat. You can raise your level of fitness by eating more nutritionally and applying the techniques of rebound exercise.

"The common denominator of all exercise is the opposition of the human body to the gravitation pull of the Earth."[1] Rebounding presents the gravitational forces of acceleration and deceleration with greater competency than any other movement. Simply, it uses vertical motion where any other exercise movement employs horizontal motion. At the bottom of the bounce, the three forces of acceleration, deceleration, and gravity come together to give you an exercise with singular power to produce a designed effect. Your result is total physiological enhancement of all cells, tissues, organs, and systems in the body.

Truly, "the most efficient, most effective form of exercise yet devised by man,"[2] is the activity delineated in *Jumping for Health.*

—Morton Walker, D.P.M.
Stamford, Connecticut

1.   Albert E. Carter. *The Miracles of Rebound Exercise.* Edmonds, WA., The National Institute of Reboundology and Health, Inc., 1979, p. 30.

2.   Ibid., p. 44.

Definition and Disclaimer

Although the apparatus used to perform rebounding aerobics looks like a miniature trampoline, it is not. Erroneously, some people have labeled the rebounding device a "mini-trampoline" when the dictionary and the manufacturers of trampolines say otherwise. A mini-trampoline is a small springy fabric platform connected to a frame which surface is set diagonally so as to allow an acrobat, gymnast, or circus performer to run, bounce, and be catapulted into the air; thus, providing enough altitude to perform intricate stunts or tricks before landing on a crash pad. The mini-trampoline is considered dangerous by professional trampolinists if used for vertical jumping as is performed in rebounding.

The word "Rebounder" is the trademark name of a rebound unit formerly manufactured by the Trimway Corporation in Seattle, Washington. Therefore, it cannot be used generically.

In this book, we refer to the rebounding device as a rebound exercise unit. This is a designated generic term applied to all the rebounding devices whether they be square, rectangular, round, polygonal, oval, or any other shape. A rebound exercise unit has certain characteristics that distinguish it from any other type of exercise equipment.

1. The height of the springy mat is set six to twelve inches from the ground.

2. The mat lies parallel with the ground.

3. The mat fabric is designed for bounding and rebounding in one place.

4. The rebound unit is not created for performing

tricks; its exclusive purpose is for exercise.

5. Anyone can use it and gymnastic expertise is unnecessary.

6. The rebound exercise unit is safe.

The rebound unit has been praised for its therapeutic value. Many people have testified to the health benefits they've received from its use. A number of case histories, in fact, are cited in this book illustrating how the rebounding device has been helpful to relieve pain, swelling and certain health problems. Yet, we wish to caution against letting rebounding equipment become any kind of substitute for proper medical attention. In other words, don't let rebounding aerobics become a replacement for competent medical advice.

We also warn you about placing too much emphasis on rebounding as the only form of exercise engaged in. Watch out that you fail to perform other movements for the sheer joy of using your muscles and the need to accomplish work. The main thing is to exercise. Keep your body in motion when feasible.

Nothing written in *Jumping for Health* should be construed as prescribing therapeutically for any health problem. The rebound unit is not a medical instrument; but where it is applied as such in this book, a health authority is cited or quoted as making the recommendation.

We do believe our recommendations are excellent holistic procedures that will aid the user in the prevention of disease; however, and toward this end we heartily suggest employment of the rebound unit.

1

Everyone Can Use Instant Aerobics

A 42-year-old desk clerk in Atlantic City, New Jersey, named Harry Malvin, viewed with alarm the size of his steadily increasing paunch. He became an early, if aging, convert of the fitness generation and took up jogging in 1976 before the sport became really popular. But Harry recently gave it up when his arches began to fall, his back suffered chronic pain, his various joints constantly ached, and his conscience no longer cried out for redemption of his sedentary sins. He's decided to look at himself in the mirror now only from the neck up. His returned paunch is being ignored.

Still, ex-jogger Malvin continues to buy and wear jogging suits and running shoes — stunning royal blue with white racing stripes that imply speed and utility. He wears out these outfits, he admits — in the seat — for he dresses in them to do nothing more than watch TV. He also wears them for walking the dog, gambling in Atlantic City casinos, strolling through shopping malls, and doing different chores around the house such as taking out the garbage.

Indeed, as an ex-jock, Harry Malvin is once again

in the vanguard of a national movement. He's among the first to stop running and start sitting. Living rooms all over this land are slowly filling now with retired joggers, faded exercise freaks, failed tennis players, previous bicycle enthusiasts, and former swimmers who find it just too much trouble to leave their homes to run through the streets, do calisthenics on a gymnasium floor, stroke balls across a tennis court, push pedals along the roads, or dive into local YW/YMCA pools.

The fitness craze that once had filled sidewalks, gymnasiums, tennis courts, bicycle paths, and swimming pools seems to have peaked at the start of the 1980s. The leveling off of fitness is creating a new subclass of people who still believe they could benefit from exercise but refuse to invest time in expending the required energy. A trade magazine for merchants who sell exercise paraphernalia, *The Sporting Goods Dealer,* in July 1979, had surveyed 40,000 American families, and reported that more than 15,000 of them, or 38 percent, were engaged in regular "general exercise." Six months later, the magazine took the same survey again and found only 12,000 families, or 30 percent, still exercising.

This survey tends to indicate that the hordes of raquetball exponents, Sunday morning baseball players, handball enthusiasts, and other participants in sports who were in pursuit of trim waists and unclogged arteries are now losing interest and having members drop from their ranks. Instead, bar stools, easy chairs, and card tables are now being occupied more. This subclass of people may continue to wear jock clothing, like Harry Malvin, but they get no closer to actual exercise than the television game of the week.

Figures from the National Sporting Goods Association also confirm a slackening of interest in participant sports. They show that tennis racket sales dropped from 8.3 million in 1977 to 4.9 million in 1978. Backpacks for hiking and camping went from 1.8 million sales in 1974 to 1.4 million in 1978. Sleeping bag sales dipped from 7.7 million in 1973 to 4.5 million in 1978. Bicycling is down 7 percent. Such staple participant sports as basketball, bowling, golf, baseball, football, and hunting also dropped during the last three years.

A physical fitness survey conducted by pollster Louis Harris and Associates for the Perrier industrial group in March 1978 also came to the conclusion that boom sports like swimming, hiking, bicycling, and tennis were falling off. He found that 85 percent of our population prefer to be armchair spectators. Jogging, which had mushroomed so suddenly in 1977 also has diminishing participants. The Harris poll's most interesting finding was that, while 59 percent of the adults said they engaged in physical activity, only 15 percent were "highly active." They did 306 minutes of exercise per week. Just 16 percent were "moderately active," doing 204 minutes weekly; 28 percent were "less active" with a maximum 150 minutes each week. The balance of 41 percent of Americans don't engage in regular forms of exercise in any way.

When Lou Harris asked people how likely they were to take up a new type of activity within the next year, only 18 percent said they were "very likely." In contrast, 42 percent were "very unlikely." Asked why they did not exercise more, they most commonly cited lack of time, inconvenience, procrastination, laziness, and too much trouble to travel to the location of their potential exercise activities.

Among the arguments most frequently cited as reasons not to exercise was the wrong-headed concern that "too much exercising can enlarge the heart, and this is bad when you stop exercising." This incorrect statement was given by 32 percent of the nonactives and 26 percent of the actives.

Another argument put forth by many — 32 percent — was that "these fads about physical fitness come and go, and I'm not impressed by the current emphasis on it."

Americans are split on the question of whether they

are getting enough exercise. Among those who do participate in sports activities, 51 percent feel they still do not get enough exercise, and 48 percent believe that they do. Among the non-actives, 48 percent are convinced that their daily routine will by itself provide enough exercise, while another 48 percent believe that it won't.

Most people who don't exercise say they don't have enough time, as we mentioned, an explanation given by 47 percent. Other obstacles to exercise are health considerations, stated by 19 percent; family responsibilities, 19 percent; the weather, 15 percent; no interest, 11 percent; and laziness, 7 percent.

However, having available time is truly not the key factor. Both the active and non-active segments of the population have approximately the same amount of leisure time available — about twenty-four hours a week.

A doctor's advice would be the strongest motivation for physical activity, according to 43 percent of the non-actives. Other factors mentioned were nicer weather, 18 percent; influence of family, 13 percent; four-day work week, 11 percent; more facilities, 10 percent; influence of friends, 10 percent. Nearly one in four — 23 percent — said that nothing would be likely to get them to engage in physical activity.

Women had been getting involved in sports and athletics at a distinctly more rapid rate than men, according to that 1978 Harris study. For example, 73 percent of all women runners had taken up the sport from 1976 to 1978, when among male runners only 53 percent had begun it in those past two years. Other sports that had been drawing women at substantial rates included tennis, softball, golf, and calisthenics, but this is not the case anymore.

It's obvious that the bloom is faded from the fad of exercising unless something new and dramatic comes along to provide a fast, fun way to health and fitness. What might this new something be?

Rebounding with the Rebound Unit

The National Institute of Reboundology and Health Inc., now located at 717 West Milford, Suite 103, Glendale, California 91203; telephone (818) 547-1513 reports that thousands of people a day are being turned on to using the new, at-home or at-work exercising apparatus known as a rebound device. The Institute's research goes back to 1975 when "rebounding" devices were first broadly introduced to the American public. The prediction is that this form of exercising will easily surpass jogging and running in popularity by 1990. And in the year 2000, most people in industrialized Western countries will have taken a turn on a rebounding-type apparatus. Many will own it for home, workplace, or areas of leisure, and almost all these owners will use the machine for achieving what might be labeled "instant aerobics."

Instant aerobics can now be engaged in the climate-controlled privacy of home, office, factory, classroom, on shipboard, even in an airliner, and, of course, outdoors—just anywhere and anytime of day or night.

Right now, even as we retreat from the exercising popularity of the 1970s, 60 million Americans are overweight and under exercised. Another 53 million have high blood pressure. Being fat, soft and hypertensive leaves these unfortunate people prone to hernia, back trouble, cancer, heart attack, stroke, and other health problems. Indeed, degenerative diseases such as cancer, heart attack, and stroke are the three biggest killers in this country. The main reason? Technology has taken away the need for people to exercise. (Poor nutrition is the second main reason.)

The odd thing is — most people in bad shape recognize the poor physical condition they're confronting. They want to be in better health and fitness, but the effort to attain this state seems too much of a burden, as we have already pointed out. They simply hate strenuous exercise. The boom in physical fitness programs continues to find popularity among the few, compared to the vast numbers who need them. In truth, after a heavy Sunday dinner and a few beers or soft drinks in front of the television set, it's common for the out-of-shape individual to vow, "I'll restart my exercising Monday morning." The vow is seldom kept.

The real circumstance is that this person just doesn't want to get up early, or drag in after work, and go through the boring and tiring calisthenics. They may hurt!

But suppose the non-active person had the ability to exercise in a gentle, enjoyable way — non-harmful muscular movements that encourage a harmony in health. He would want this, wouldn't he? Wouldn't you?

The bounce of rebounding provides you with the freedom of moving, turning, twisting, kicking, and stretching the body without pain and performed at your own pace.

Rebounding is bouncing from gentle to vigorous in a vertical action that is anti-gravity, as on a pogo stick, a diving board, or when a child bounces on the bed. Performing on a giant trampoline is a rebound action creating an aerobic effect. Using the rebounding device is a simplified and safer version of giant-size trampolining.

The difference between a big trampoline and the tiny, short-legged device is that no attempt to bounce high or do any gymnastic tricks is made on the mini-model. It allows numerous bodily movements at this low, safe level. If you wish, you can hold on for support. The effect of bouncing is the same. It's the rare person who doesn't enjoy the movements of rebounding. Children just love the feeling, and adults crave the aerobic benefits (described in detail in the next chapter). Now they have the ability to acquire aerobic benefits easily, conveniently, without risk, in a painless way, and with minimal effort. It's the newly invented way to get instant aerobics by bouncing that everyone can use.

The rebounding device is either round, rectangular, square, polygonal, or some other shape and approximately thirty-six inches in diameter. It rests on four to eight legs, six to nine inches high. Using this rebound unit definitely fills the requirement for a new, fast, fun way to health and fitness. Rebounding is so easy, it overcomes laziness and provides a general sense of well being. Those who rebound find themselves able to work without tiring, sleeping better, eating more nutritiously, and feeling less tense. It's not just psychological, because the exercise of bouncing up and down against gravity but without trauma to the musculoskeletal system is the most beneficial exercise yet developed by man. Rebounding has proven itself as the perfect exercise for both sexes, every age, for the most physically adept athlete, and especially for a handicapped person who uses the device in a certain way tailored to his or her needs.

If you want to reduce fat and cellulite on your legs, thighs, arms, and hips; increase your agility and improve your sense of balance; add strength and firmness to muscles all over your body; rehabilitate a physical injury; provide an aerobic effect for the heart routinely and periodically; inhale more air by increasing lung capacity; improve vision by strengthening eye muscles; exercise the internal organs in the way no other motion can manage; generally rejuvenate a tired body — in a living room, a basement, a garage, at the office — naturally, pleasurably, and scientifically, read on about this unique form of movement that we call "rebounding aerobics." It is aimed at the overall fitness and health of your body.

Nancy Martin's Experience with Rebounding

Nancy M. Martin of Goodville, Pennsylvania experienced a number of physical improvements from engaging in rebound exercise. Mrs. Martin, who is now seventy-seven years young, had suffered from chronic disequilibrium, a problem of the middle-ear, that she remembers having as far back as 1946. Then, she felt she might fall while singing with an acapella choir at Greenwood, Delaware. "Maintaining my balance while standing on the stage was exceedingly difficult," she recalled in a letter she wrote to us for publication.

"Through the years, sometimes my having poor equilibrium was more pronounced than other times. Standing still, unsupported, or when bending over, is when I felt out of balance. But as soon as I began walking or moving in some way I was all right. Often, while waiting in line at the bank, standing in a cafeteria, or even holding a conversation with someone and seeing no support available, it was not only annoying to me, but almost beyond endurance to bear. As I hung clothes on the wash line, I'd shake from my knees down like a leaf fluttering in the wind. But exercise, such as walking a few steps, would help me get balanced again."

For over thirty years, Mrs. Martin accepted this disequilibrium problem as part of everyday living. Several times she fell on her front lawn from merely picking up a few leaves.

While attending a lecture given by C. Samuel West, D.N., an exponent of jumping for health, Mrs. Martin saw one of these rebound units for the first time. "I thought I could never use one," wrote the woman, and she told this to Frank Angelo, a former demonstrator of rebound exercise. "That's all the more reason why you need one," she quotes him as replying. The woman was convinced she would never acquire a rebound unit for herself.

"At that time, had I attempted to stand on one unsupported I'd have screamed, feeling like I was falling off a house roof. Would you believe it? — I changed my mind, bought one and was never sorry. Today I'm able to stand and do exercises without any support most of the time, but not yet 100%. I'm beginning to see a light at the end of the tunnel."

For instance, her left hip, which was injured in 1942, had caused sporadic discomfort many times since, with medication helping only for short periods. Yet, in 1977, the year she purchased her rebounding device, the hip trouble just stopped after she began using it. "I no longer have this discomfort," said Mrs. Martin, "and am convinced that rebounding took care of the problem."

Then, she used the gentle bouncing exercise to strengthen her eyes against cataracts. Cataracts? Let's let Mrs. Martin tell her own story. "Several years ago the ophthalmologist told me I was starting with cataracts. It nearly floored me. He sensed my utter surprise and said that it goes with the process of aging. I didn't feel old enough for that yet. Still, several years later during another visit to the eye doctor, he told me my cataracts weren't making any progress and, indeed, were getting worse.

"In February 1980, I purchased a narrated cassette tape on visual therapy with fifteen exercises described. Vision therapy performed on the rebounding apparatus is a program introduced by Albert E. Carter and narrated by Paul Herlinger. I listened to the instructions and performed the visual exercises faithfully.

"One of the exercises is a fine print card drill with several paragraphs, each one a smaller print, in turn. Purposely I refrained from reading the fine print while wearing my glasses so that I couldn't memorize any of the words. And, I couldn't read one word of the paragraphs without wearing them. To my complete surprise, in less than three weeks I could read the first three paragraphs without glasses (although the print is too fine to read the lines for an overly long time). As my eye muscles improve, I'll probably need to have my lenses changed to weaker prescriptions and maybe decrease their strength repeatedly. The gentle bounce of rebounding suggested with these visual exercises has been beneficial to my eyes."

Further Body Function Benefits

Mrs. Nancy Martin's rebounding experience is not at all surprising when you consider how regular exercise improves body functions. John A. Friedrich, M.D. of Duke University, writing in the *Journal of Physical Education,* says that moving the muscles, especially the large leg muscles as done in rebounding, aids blood circulation exceedingly. Dr. Friedrich stated, "the combination of the large leg muscles massaging the blood back to the heart along with the effect of the diaphragmatic action very significantly enhances the total circulatory efficiency, and in the process, minimizes the stress put on the heart, inasmuch as the leg muscles and diaphragm act as auxiliary hearts by assisting in blood flow."[1]

In the chapters that follow, we will go into detail on the physiological benefits of rebounding and other endurance exercises. In this chapter, we'll just briefly alert you to some of the more significant physiological improvements occurring from your overloading the muscles with rebounding aerobics, as you go on to practice regularly.

CARDIORESPIRATORY IMPROVEMENTS

The individual who uses his rebound unit regularly can expect to experience some of the following cardiorespiratory changes listed by Dr. Friedrich:

(1) He or she will increase vital capacity. This means that the lungs will be able to handle more oxygen and

---

[1] John A. Friedrich. "How jogging improves body functions." *Journal of Physical Education* (May-June 1970), p. 124.

the ventilation potential of the body will increase.

(2) More functioning capillaries will become available in the lungs and thereby more potential for oxygen absorption.

(3) A greater capacity for incurring an oxygen debt will come about. The rebounding person will be able to repay an oxygen debt to the cells, tissues, and organs more rapidly, and there will be faster gaseous exchange within the lungs.

(4) The increased flexibility of the chest wall which occurs from movement of the entire torso will aid respiratory function.

(5) Latent capillaries in various body tissues will open up to minimize peripheral circulatory resistance as well as providing more effective tissue oxygenation.

(6) During the actual rebounding period the rate and depth of respiration increases as does the rate and force of the heart beat. However, the resting heart rate will decrease and the resting blood pressure, if elevated, will also tend to decrease.

CARDIOVASCULAR IMPROVEMENTS

Not the least of body functioning benefits take place from alterations in the cardiovascular system as a whole when regular and sustained rebounding aerobics are made part of everyday routine. Dr. Friedrich provided some examples:

(1) The red blood cell count as well as the blood hemoglobin tend to increase.

(2) Small blood vessels of the skin and muscles open up with an engorgement of blood streaming to these moving organs.

(3) The heart stroke volume builds up to its optimum amount. This means that more blood can be pumped with each stroke of the heart, which in turn lowers the resting heart rate, as mentioned. The heart muscle thus works more efficiently.

(4) An increased number of functioning capillaries

grows into the cardiac muscle itself (and also the other muscles in motion around the body) as collatoral circulation. The result is that more oxygen is carried to the cardiac muscle.

(5) Besides collateral circulation, the openings of existing coronary arteries widen more.

(6) Elevated blood cholesterol and glyceride levels tend to lower.

(7) High density lipoproteins that prevent heart attack build up.

(8) A high blood viscosity that might bring on blood clots is lessened. The blood gets thinner from rebound exercise.

MISCELLANEOUS IMPROVEMENTS

Besides the foregoing advantages to entire body systems, various other general physiological values are suggested by Dr. Friedrich as coming from an aerobic exercise like rebounding. He listed a few:

(1) The cortisone hormone balance of the adrenal glands evens out, and the adrenals themselves are conditioned and fortified so that more severe stresses may be handled adequately.

(2) The supply of cortisone required for body homeostasis is kept at its optimum thus minimizing calcium loss from the blood stream, and storage organs.

(3) Metabolism is enhanced and there is better absorption of nutrients from food intake.

(4) The processes of digestion, appetite, and elimination all get noticeably better.

(5) The tendency for constipation, kidney stones, or diabetes is lessened.

(6) Fatty degenerations of the body, especially those areas around the heart, the lungs, the blood vessels and the brain often seen in sedentary individuals, almost cease their formation.

The relatively short time that it takes to rebound daily, perhaps five minutes to twenty minutes to forty minutes per rebounding session, depending on your condition and motivation, will be time well spent for acquiring the important benefits we have already delineated. There's no doubt that the more you use your rebounding device, the more you'll bring your body back to nearyouthfulness.

Bounding away for the betterment of the human body was an idea that germinated in the minds of the original developers of the rebounding industry. They have studied the sport of trampolining and transposed it into the science of *reboundology — the newest means for men and women to acquire health, strength, physical fitness, mental relaxation, and emotional stability.

A Short History of *Reboundology

The science of bouncing up and down in a vertical plane without performing tricks is *reboundology. It was a natural derivation from trampolining, which the *Guinness Book of World Records* describes as beginning about 1911. The Nissen Corporation, under the leadership of George Nissen, had been the major force behind the promotion of the trampolining sport.

The rebound unit was first created in a crude form by a man named Ed Russell about 1938. He brought his pilot model to Victor Green who was then a public relations counselor and advertising agent. Russell lost interest afterward, but Green became intrigued with the device, added a number of improvements, and filed for a patent. He held the invention patent pending for twelve years so as not to expose his changes to other potential manufacturers. Eventually the United States Patent Office forced Green to reveal his methods by publishing them in the public documents and issued him a patent number 3892403, July 1, 1975. He became president of the Tri-Flex Manufacturing, Inc. located in South Houston, Texas. The company built a rectangular rebounding device 45 inches long by 33 inches wide, and other size units.

*See page viii

The Leffler Company of Portland, Oregon built rebound units as therapeutic tools for vision correction. Vision therapists employed the small rebound device to strengthen eye muscles, beginning about forty years ago. Square commercial units sold as exercising devices were made by the Trampa Company in Houston, Texas.

A designer of engineered devices, Ed Anderson of Las Vegas, Nevada, built the first round units for rebounding. He ran production for the Vital Corporation, Incorporated under the laws of Nevada. The first public presentation of rebounding exercises was in 1975 in Seattle, Washington. Gerald Hinkle, president of the Trimway Corporation of Seattle, conducted his Rebounder demonstration in a Ramada Inn conference room.

Rebound exercise might be considered to have become a science and an established industry when Albert E. Carter, a skilled trampolinist on the giant, sport model trampolines, published a booklet describing the physiology of "reboundology," a word he coined and trademarked. *Rebound to Better Health*, issued in 1977, introduced the reader and sportsperson to this new form of exercise.

In 1979, *The Miracles of Rebound Exercise*, his first full-sized book, was published by the National Institute of Reboundology and Health, Inc. (NIRH) of which Carter is still president. *Miracles* gave a detailed overview of rebounding, including history, theory, charts, graphs, pictures, and testimonials of users. In it, Carter described rebounding, as "the most efficient, effective form of exercise yet devised by man," but he also admitted it to be a form of human activity that was the least understood.[2]

By 1977, there were at least five U.S. manufacturers competing for the developing rebound exercise market. With new industrial formation came some of the typical business practices: design theft, personal endorsements of rebound units, mass media advertising, multi-level marketing, foreign competition, and finally price cutting which

---

[2]Albert E. Carter. *Rebound to Better Health*. (Lynnwood, Washington: Paco's Press, 1977), p. vii.

inevitably ended with quality cutting of the devices being manufactured.

There were over 100 known American manufacturers building rebound devices of all shapes and sizes in 1981, when department stores and mass merchandisers such as Montgomery Ward and Company, Sears Roebuck and Company, and J.C. Penney Company, Inc. began offering the rebound device manufacturers huge orders if they would make the individual units inexpensive enough.

More than 1,500,000 rebound devices were sold in the United States in 1983 alone. Observing all of this business activity, the foreign manufacturers were soon stealing the market from the Americans, forcing many domestic manufacturers out of business. However, the foreigners knew nothing about rebound exercise, although they did understand how to incorporate cheaper materials and cheaper labor. An astounding $72 million was spent by consumers for the purchase of rebounding devices during 1984, but the units proved to be inferior. Many of them were pitched into the trash by disgusted consumers when the device's springs broke, the legs broke off, or the mat split. The original dedicated U.S. manufacturers received only 13 percent of this vast sales volume, much of which was taken at a loss through the closeouts of merchandise.

It was sad to see the disintegration of a budding industry. For example, the National Institute of Reboundology and Health had been the main supplier of literature for the industry. As the main manufacturers went out of business and since the cheap units being sold didn't furnish literature, the NIRH lost almost all of its literature sales. The Institute temporarily closed its doors.

Al Carter accepted an engagement in Australia where he gave seminars and media interviews on rebound exercise. While there, he was approached by Peter Daetweiler to come to Hong Kong to help in the selling of rebounding to the Government of that British colony. Rebounding was recommended as the prime exercise for the police and fire departments in Hong Kong. Before he did so, the units available on the market were tested by Daetweiler and Carter. It was decided that a rebound device had to be designed that could withstand the constant use of many users without failing. Carter was assigned three engineers to help him do the designing. In two weeks he accomplished the task, and the Hong Kong Government agreed to acquire 20,000 units of Carter's newly designed rebounding device.

It was a functional, durable machine named "the Dynabound." It became well-accepted in Asia. The Dynabound was made round, because a circle is the strongest of all geometric structures in a single plane. It was built nine inches off the ground so that a 300-pound man could not hit the floor while bouncing as high as possible. Yet, Dynabound was low enough so that a six-foot, two-inch person would not hit his head on a standard ceiling. The mat was made of Dupont Permatron™. It won't stretch and does outlast the latter three materials by three to one.

The new jumping device had springs made of a more durable number 80 carbon steel alloy. The springs were connected to hardened bolts through the frame instead of into holes drilled into the frame. Frame-drilled holes can wear out the frame in 36 places within a short time period. In contrast, using bolts should see the frame last forever. The legs were made to fold with spring to hold them in place because the screw-on-type legs can get lost or the threads may strip with ease.

Since space is at a premium in Hong Kong, the solid circle frame was cut in half and hinged with a special offset hinge that locks in the open position. The folded unit is small enough to fit in the trunk of an automobile, the back of a closet, under the bed, or in the overhead luggage bin in most airplanes. This new unit was and still is being manufactured in Taiwan to keep costs down. But its entire manufacturing process is being done under the supervision of NIRH personnel.

2

The Aerobic Effect of Rebounding

While Kenneth H. Cooper, M.D., M.P.H., author of *Aerobics* and founder of the Institute for Aerobics Research in Dallas, Texas, is the acknowledged inventor of the modern day aerobic concept, Maimonides, who lived in the twelfth century, advocated another form of aerobics: exercise to the point of breathlessness.

Dr. Cooper has developed and made famous a point system which measures the effectiveness of various kinds of exercise. He arrived at his system in 1968, before rebounding aerobics even existed.[1] Indeed, his system was arrived at seven years prior to the time the rebound unit had been manufactured for wide consumer distribution. Still, this physician had good insight into the value of jumping, skipping, and bounding up and down against gravity, because he put rope jumping at the top of his list of beneficial aerobic exercises.

Cooper assigned skipping rope three points and indicated that jumping for ten minutes is equivalent to

---

[1]Kenneth H. Cooper. *Aerobics.* (New York: M. Evan and Co., 1968), p. 29.

skiing thirty minutes, vigorously dancing the hustle for forty minutes, or playing two sets of singles tennis for forty minutes. Other scientific evidence has reported that jumping rope for ten minutes is as effective in conditioning the body as approximately thirty minutes of fast jogging.

Rebounding on a rebound unit is practically the same as jumping rope except you don't get the jarring effect to the ankles, knees, and low back that you do from hitting the solid ground. You can swing your arms while bouncing on the rebounding device's stretched cushion. It provides an **aerobic effect** or **training response** for the entire body, including the internal organs.

This aerobic or training response is the whole goal of endurance exercise. It increases the efficiency of the lungs so that they process more air. It enhances the functioning of the heart muscle to grow stronger and pump more blood with each stroke. This reduces the number of heavy heart beats necessary. A conditioned person may have a resting heart rate twenty beats per minute slower than a deconditioned person. He saves 10,000 beats in one night's sleep. His heart lasts longer from working less.

The aerobic effect increases the number and size of the blood vessels that carry the blood around the body. From rebounding aerobics, you acquire a greater total blood volume to deliver more oxygen to the cells of all tissues and organs.

To repeat, the theory of aerobics is that improvement of the functioning of the heart, lungs, and blood vessels through exercise, in this case by rebounding, will optimize the body's utilization of oxygen. For you, this will result in a lower coronary risk profile and better general health. The longer you do an exercise and the faster you work at it, the greater will be the endurance you work up to.

In an interview with Dr. Kenneth Cooper, he said that once people start engaging in aerobic exercises on a regular basis, what has them continue diligently is more than increased physical capacity. "It's the psychological improvement, too, the fact that they do feel better," he said. "They have a more positive outlook, more enthusiasm, and are more productive with their daily activities. A person who is physically fit gains a whole new zest for life that he doesn't have when he's not physically fit. When I lecture on this topic, I tell people, 'You will feel better.' Probably 90 percent of followers of my aerobics program have told me, when I asked what motivates them, that they continue exercising because it makes them feel better.

"Sometimes, people also tell me they don't see the need to exercise because they already feel good. I say, 'Do you really? How good could you feel? Do you know? You don't unless you have tried exercise.'

"That new zest for life, the psychological factor, is what I believe has propagated this whole health movement to use exercise as a major modality of preventive medicine."[2]

Aerobic training wasn't always accepted by the public, and especially not by establishment medical practitioners. The ideas Dr. Cooper currently expounds at first met with opposition from the orthodox medical profession as a whole. "Twenty years ago, I was considered a quack," he said. "Now, I'm getting invitations to become a visiting professor at medical schools all over the country. The Mayo Clinic has invited me to lecture, which I think is quite an honor. That's the sort of acceptance aerobic exercise is getting now.

"The American Medical Association has been supportive. Its view is that what we need in America is a lot more preventive medicine and a whole lot less treatment medicine. The cost of treatment medicine is too high, and as we become more sophisticated in our diagnostic techniques from a treatment standpoint, the price just continues to keep going up," added Dr. Cooper.

---

[2]Robert C. Anderson. "The self-help way to health." *Success Unlimited* (March 1988), pp. 15-17.

"For example, about 200,000 coronary bypass procedures were performed last year *(220,000 in 1988)*. It is possible that some of those people could have been treated successfully through a program of aerobic conditioning, with results almost as good as those from bypass surgery and at a tiny fraction of the cost. So to control the escalating cost of health care in the future, we must try to prevent problems, not only treat them," the aerobics inventor concluded.[3]

The use of your rebounding device will give you a physical training response the same as or better than certain accepted aerobic exercises such as jogging, rowing, swimming, racquet sports, cycling, hiking, timed calisthenics, or any other exertion you undertake to combine fitness and activity to breathe in more oxygen and have a conditioning effect on the heart and lungs. Furthermore, the muscles and blood vessels improve in tone, fat weight changes to lean weight, and endurance increases.

Overall, the training response from aerobic activity on the rebound unit increases maximal oxygen consumption by increasing the efficiency of the means of supply and delivery. In the very act of using the low device for rebounding, you improve the condition of your body, especially its most vital parts, the lungs, the heart, the blood vessels, and the body cells to build a bulwark against many forms of illness and disease.

Hearing Returns to Ethel B. Lane

Rebounding aerobics was the only treatment used by Ethel B. Lane of Seattle, Washington, age eighty-six, to restore her hearing after its loss following a fall.

In July 1979, directly after my first appearance in Seattle to lecture on "Total Health, the Holistic Alternative to Traditional Medicine that Stresses Preventive Care, Nutri-

---

[3]*Ibid.*

tion, and Treatment of the Whole Person,"[4] Mrs. Lane came forward to describe how she used rebound exercise to help her hearing return. She explained, "I attended a lecture on rebounding sponsored by Esther Brown and saw the beneficial effects of this form of exercise. I bought one of those little bouncing machines from Mrs. Brown and started using it. She recommended for me to start slowly and each day increase my time bouncing.

"In the latter part of February 1979 I had fallen, and the injury impaired my hearing," Mrs. Lane said. "I couldn't hear at all. Now my hearing is coming back to what it was before. If all people will just speak slowly, I can catch every word."

We asked, "Mrs. Lane, is rebounding the only treatment you're taking for yourself?"

"Well, I also take long walks!"

"Do you attribute the return of your hearing to rebounding, Mrs. Lane?"

"Yes, I do! I think exercise is the answer. Of course, I also try to live nutritionally — eat a lot of fresh vegetables and fruits. Now that fruits are in season my breakfast is mostly fruit."

We tried to tie her story to the lecture we had just presented: "In other words, you are living holistically — in 'total health' — and you've made rebounding a part of your life."

"Yes!" she replied.

"And do you, at age eighty-six, believe rebounding is good for any age person?"

"Absolutely, any age. There are some friends my age and younger who have come to my home and used my rebounding machine. And they've experienced a wonderful feeling when they get on it. One lady who has headaches and pain in the back of her head, I've been

---

[4]Morton Walker. *Total Health: The Holistic Alternative to Traditional Medicine that Stresses Preventive Care, Nutrition, and Treatment of the Whole Person.* (New York: Everest House, 1979).

trying to get to buy a bouncy machine for herself, because I believe it will help her get rid of the head pain the way it helped my hearing to return."

"What do you think there is in the apparatus that helps you? Why should it be restoring your hearing?"

"Exercise," she declared. "It's a form of convenient exercise. When you can't get out in the rain or are too busy to take long walks, you just jump on the thing and bounce away."

"Mrs. Lane, you know you've been speaking here into a recording machine. May we use what you have said for publication in a book?"

"Yes, you may!"

"Thank you, Mrs. Lane."

The woman is correct in pointing to rebound exercise as the source of her hearing improvement or for its employment against other forms of illness.

Every cell in the body depends on a plentiful supply of food and oxygen in the blood stream. When the blood circulatory system becomes sluggish or congested, vital nutrition and oxygen are denied the individual cells.

For Mrs. Lane, the physical trauma of her fall may have caused previous circulatory blockage in the blood vessels leading to the ears to show up suddenly. You can have up to 70 percent occlusion of the arteries without any symptoms of pathology, but stress the cardiovascular system just a little more and signs of hardening of the arteries then come on suddenly. In this elderly woman, her blood vessels, like the pipes in a city water system after many years of service, became congested. If the water system could be cleansed by some method, the usefulness and service of its pipes could be extended considerably. For Mrs. Lane's circulatory system, exercise has proved to be such a cleansing method. The bouncing motion massages the muscle walls of the blood vessels into carrying off impurities collected by the blood from the trillions of body cells, including her auditory nerve cells. Some impurities eventually broke out from the neurons innervating her hearing sense. Cellular wastes were carried away and a new supply of food and oxygen arrived in its place. (See chapter four on the lymphatic system to learn how this waste removal is accomplished.) Keeping up her rebounding action steadily restored formerly impaired hearing for Ethel B. Lane.

Cardiopulmonary Endurance Exercise

The first and most independent act we perform as human beings is to breathe. Without being attached to our mothers through the umbilical cord, each oxygen molecule we inhale becomes essential to our active tissues. They won't function without it. Brain tissue, for example, must not be deprived of oxygen or neurons will die and never be able to regenerate. The blood is the carrying medium for oxygen and many other molecules bound in chemical combinations. Thus, the cardiovascular and pulmonary systems work in unison to pull in oxygen and circulate it around the body.

Red blood cells attract oxygen molecules to themselves because of the presence of a protein, called **hemoglobin.** While a small amount of oxygen is carried in physical combination with the red blood cells, the greater portion of this life-giving gas is carried in chemical combination as **oxyhemoglobin.** The principal function of streaming red blood cells is to carry the oxygen molecule to the different active body cells and carry away the end products of metabolism, especially the waste gas, carbon dioxide.

Physiological investigations have revealed that the oxygen saturation of blood maintains itself best in a more active individual. It may retain as high as 95 percent for someone who stays moving and using his muscles in work, recreation, or just for the pleasure of exercising. An inactive person, on the other hand, can suffer from blood oxygen starvation and manifest such a state by feeling fatigued, acting lethargic, and thinking unclearly. The reason? An inadequate oxygen supply to the brain holds this organ in a malnourished condition. The brain's processes carry on strictly from being fueled by glucose and oxygen. Deprive it of either and you'll experience the symptoms we've listed — and much worse.

The answer to keeping the brain functioning well is to move around enough so that the streaming blood carries its ideal complement of oxygen — 95 percent saturation. Inadequate oxygen delivery can invariably be traced to the cardiovascular system not getting enough input from the cardiopulmonary system.

Everyone can gain from the application of a routine cardiopulmonary endurance exercise a number of times throughout the day. Such an exercise would improve the rate of oxygen delivery and the exchange of gases — of oxygen delivered into the blood stream, of carbon dioxide taken from it. All of us should exercise in accordance with Maimonides' recommendation: exercise to the point of breathlessness.

In-place running on your rebounding device for uninterrupted periods in excess of five minutes would steadily build up cardiopulmonary endurance and insure saturation of the blood with oxygen molecules. H.C. Carlson, Ph.D., an exercise physiologist and coach of basketball at the University of Pittsburgh, has proposed an excellent system of in-place running for cardiovascular-pulmonary conditioning. Run on the rebounding device for ten seconds and count the number of single foot contacts. Rest for ten seconds. Try to increase the number of single foot contacts by at least one each time you do an interval of rebound running. Rest for ten seconds between each run. See if you can keep this up for five minutes.

You'll discover that Dr. Carlson's technique is hard work, especially if you play fairly with yourself and raise your feet high with each bounce.[5]

Another reason to carry out routine cardiopul-

[5]Benjamin Ricci. *Physical and Physiological Conditioning for Men.* (Dubuque, Iowa: Wm. C. Brown Co., 1972), p. 51.

monary endurance exercises is to condition the heart muscle to increase the volume of blood it ejects per contraction. To train the heart to do this, it must be placed under a fairly constant level of stress for a given period of time, not too little and not too much. Routine employment of a cardiopulmonary endurance exercise will increase the heart's efficiency, make it stronger, and heighten its pumping capacity. You can tell if this is occurring by measuring your pulse rate for a given load of exercise. A drop in the number of beats means your heart is gaining efficiency.

How to Measure Your Heart's Efficiency

Your heart responds to **overload.** Overload is simply the extra demand placed upon it to condition the heart and get it to grow stronger. Remember, the heart is merely a muscle that reacts to a particular load placed on it, followed by a period of rest — a stress-rest sequence. This regular sequence provides cardiac training. The better sort of sequence is aerobic exercise carried out for a minimum of thirty minutes, at least three times a week, at an intensity sufficient to raise the pulse rate to a specific target zone.

Target zones vary with the individual's state of health, his age, and how fit he has kept himself. For example, a normally sedentary fifty-five-year-old person may hit a target pulse of 140 beats per minute merely from walking briskly for five minutes. A younger trained athlete may approach 140 beats per minute only after running at top speed for thirty minutes. The differences in heart rate derive from age, conditioning, heredity, nutrition, and the starting point of overall fitness. Consequently, the older, less active person must not begin with a really strenuous program of physical effort.

Rebounding would be exactly the correct form of aerobics for either individual, because he could vary his length of time on the rebound unit, the vigor of his bouncing, the types of rebounding exercise performed, and his number of rebound sessions. Feelings of comfort, breathlessness, or speed of pulse rate as one performs in his target zone are the determinants of how much bouncing he could do.

We suggest the following procedure to measure progress as your heart gains efficiency from your program of rebounding aerobics: Take your pulse rate as soon as you stop any full session of rebounding. Record the beat by placing your finger tips over the cartoid artery in the neck, just slightly to either side of the chin and press with a moderate amount of pressure. You can also check at the radial artery for the pulse in the wrist. Or, you can lay your hand over your heart, feeling for its beat. Count the number of beats in ten seconds, multiply by six, and record the rate for one minute.

Table I provides an idea of target zones for certain ages. As a person grows older, the highest heart rate which can be reached during an all-out effort tends to fall. The numerical values shown are "average"' values, but realize that one-third of the population may differ from these values.

Table I
Target Zones and Maximal Attainable Heart Rates*

Age in Years	Target Zone Beats/Minute	Maximal Attainable Beat/Minute
25	140 to 170	200
30	136 to 165	194
35	132 to 160	188
40	128 to 155	182
45	124 to 150	176
50	119 to 145	171
55	115 to 140	165
60	111 to 135	159
65	107 to 130	153

*From Lenore R. Zohman, *Beyond Diet . . . Exercise Your Way to Fitness and Heart Health* (Englewood Cliffs, NJ; CPC International, Inc., 1974), p. 15.

The cardiopulmonary training of the heart increases as you exercise regularly. Your stroke volume, the amount of blood pumped out of the heart chambers on each stroke, steadily becomes greater. You'll need less beats per minute to pump out the same amount of blood to the body as you did when you had been untrained. Soon you'll see, no doubt, that this training response comes into play anytime you're forced into some form of exertion.

You'll be able to notice your heart has acquired a training response in about six to fifteen weeks, depending on how faithfully you have used your rebound unit and also depending on your prior state of health. The greatest and fastest improvement in heart health will be witnessed from engaging in rebounding aerobics for at least one session of forty minutes or more a day, a minimum of five days out of seven. We suggest you bounce for this length of time using a variety of rebound exercises that we'll describe in chapter ten. Moreover, you can make the time pass quickly by diverting your attention with bouncing while watching television, listening to music, performing visual training exercises, or talking on the telephone.

Perhaps you will notice the paradox here, where the best way to lower the resting heart rate is to make it beat faster during prolonged periods of exercise. The extra exertion strengthens the heart so that it performs more efficiently at lower rates.

The heart is strengthened two ways during exercise, first by improving the quality of the muscle itself, and second by increasing the coordination of the fibers as they wring blood out of the heart during each beat.

The heart works something like a wet sponge. Its cells are similar to a sponge's cells saturated with liquid. Compress the sponge tightly and uniformly, and you'll extract the maximum amount of liquid from it. In the same way, the muscle fibers squeeze the heart cells to pull out the maximum quantity of blood lodged in chambers around which the cells are formed. The heart's muscle fibers need training, like any athlete's muscles. When they're worked less and get lazy, they tend to be uncoordinated during those times they are forced to work. Some of the fibers become sluggish, so others must work harder and more frequently in order to move the blood back around in required quantities.

The overload we spoke of earlier acts to condition the heart's muscle fibers by pushing its rate to a level a little higher than usual for longer than a few minutes. You don't have to be a marathon runner to lower your resting heart rate about ten beats a minute. Any training you do on a regular basis that puts a slight overload on your heart will accomplish the job. Engaging in rebounding aerobics is the ideal way for almost every person, trained and untrained alike. The lower heart rate rebounding aerobics finally accomplishes for the individual is the barometer of a more efficiently working heart muscle. It lets you feel more alive, less fatigued, with an almost unlimited capacity for activity.

Exercise Helps to Dissolve Blood Clots

A series of studies performed at Duke University, and published in the May 1, 1980 issue of the *New England Journal of Medicine*, have added to the growing body of evidence that physical fitness can reduce the risk of developing and dying of heart and blood vessel diseases. Researchers have found that regular, vigorous exercise such as rebounding aerobics, improves a person's ability to dissolve blood clots, an effect that could have life saving benefits.

Led by a cardiologist, R. Sanders Williams, M.D., the Duke University researchers measured the biochemical response to a blockage of veins in sixty-nine healthy adults aged twenty-five to sixty-nine before and after they participated in a ten-week physical conditioning program. The investigators used a newly developed radioactive technique to detect the release of substances into the blood that helps dissolve blood clots.

This clot-dissolving ability, known as **fibrinolytic activity,** is normally called into play by the body when something, usually a clot, closes off a blood vessel. The greater the fibrinolytic response, the faster the clot is dissolved, reducing the chances of serious medical consequences from the blockage.

The persons in the study exercised under supervision three times a week; enough to raise their heart rate to 70 to 85 percent of its maximum ability to beat (see Table I). Before the program began and after ten weeks of participation, the medical researchers temporarily simulated a clot in the subjects by blowing up a blood pressure cuff fitted around the arm until it closed off the arm veins.

An analysis of blood samples from the closed-off veins showed that at the end of the exercise program, the blood contained significantly more fibrinolytic activity than before exercise. This improved ability to dissolve clots was noted even though the participants did not significantly change other factors that increase heart attack risk, such as cigarette smoking, weight or blood cholesterol levels, and exposure to external pollution.

Obviously, the publication of these series of studies provides an additional explanation for the recovery of hearing for Mrs. Ethel B. Lane, whom we have already described. Her rebounding aerobics probably produced fibrinolytic activity in the blocked arteries nourishing her auditory sense. The result is that any clots present became dissolved and allowed blood to flow through to nourish her ears. In effect, Mrs. Lane gives her hearing a treatment every time she goes for a long walk or jumps on her "bouncy machine."

In an editorial in the same issue of the *New England Journal of Medicine,* Ralph S. Paffenbarger, M.D., an epidemiologist at the California State Department of Health, who had completed the first demonstration showing physical activity participated in for at least three hours a week allowed for fewer heart attacks among Harvard alumni than those who did not exercise, made an observation. He noted that the Duke study we've just cited "is one of a number of investigations that bolster with physiological evidence the so-called "circumstantial" case for exercise as an essential protective element in human health." He added, "It is no longer difficult to accept the view that exercise has a direct and favorable association with processes important to cardiovascular health."

In an earlier investigation of 3,686 San Francisco longshoremen, Dr. Paffenbarger and his associates did a statistical analysis of union medical records from 1951 to 1973. These longshoremen were between the ages of thirty-five and seventy-four. The investigating doctors found that taking it easy on the job was as potent a risk as smoking one or more packs of cigarettes a day. In the twenty-two years of the period studied, 395 men died from heart attacks; forty-nine of them had jobs requiring hard work (lifting, shoving, pushing heavy material) and seventy-one were in middle-energy jobs; the rest of the men (275) worked in light jobs — the equivalent of office work — even though fewer than half of all longshoremen do such jobs. Men between thirty-five and fifty-five in the most strenuous jobs had the fewest fatal heart attacks. They were also much less likely to die within one hour of an attack (the sudden-death syndrome).

Dr. Paffenbarger believes that if all the longshoremen had worked strenuously, deaths from heart attacks might have been reduced by half (194 fewer heart attacks). He is uncertain whether hard work triggers some sort of protection against heart attacks or whether inactivity in itself leads to an increased risk. He and his colleagues concluded that, particularly among younger men, the relationships among exercise, hard work, and a healthy heart are too strong to ignore.[6]

---

[6]Jody Gaylin. "Hard work and healthy hearts," *Psychology Today* (July 1977), pg. 25.

Physical Activity Increases HDL

In March 1979, we attended a medical conference in New Orleans sponsored by the American Heart Association (AHA). One of the physicians presenting a paper was Richard Remington, M.D., dean of the University of Michigan School of Public Health, who stated flat out that physical activity has a protective effect against heart disease, and it does this in a specific way. His description matched what we have already described.

William L. Haskell, M.D. of Stanford University School of Medicine explained at the same AHA meeting that moderate activity — for example, rebounding for ten minutes daily — increases the amount of high-density lipoproteins (HDL) in the blood. These proteins seem to remove cholesterol from arteries and encourage its excretion. People who suffer heart attacks tend to have very low levels of HDL, and those with high levels are far less prone to heart disease than the average person.

"Physical activity seems to be the best way to increase HDL levels," Dr. Haskell said. His study of 4,600 men and women showed that exercise itself raised high density lipoprotein levels after taking into account differences between active and inactive individuals in smoking and drinking habits and amount of body fat. He reported that exercise increased this type of lipoprotein that is naturally higher in women than in men and is believed to be one factor explaining the relative immunity of women to heart attacks.

Furthermore, independent research by L. Howard Hartley, M.D., confirmed Dr. Haskell's finding. Dr. Hartley is Director of Exercise at Beth Israel Hospital in Boston and Associate Professor of Medicine, Harvard Medical School. He said, "Exercise can have a direct effect on blood fats," and studies have shown that "people who exercise regularly reduce their levels of serum cholesterol and serum triglycerides."

His studies also showed that exercise increases levels

of HDL fractions of cholesterol and "all of these effects of exercise are expected to have a favorable effect on cardiovascular health maintenance."

Dr. Hartley also stated that when people engage in regular physical activity, they have a reduction in their systolic blood pressure level, and the amount of reduction tends to correlate with the level of the blood pressure to begin with. "People with higher levels of blood pressure to begin with show a greater reduction than do those with lower or normal pressures,'" he explained. "In fact, if they have pressures on the low side, exercise conditioning does not change their pressure level at all." Thus, rebounding aerobics tends to lower elevated blood pressure.

Do Heart Attacks Hit Healthy Exercisers?

In chapter one, we pointed out an erroneous belief held by non-exercising people that regular physical activity enlarges the heart and may even bring on heart disease. Often they'll point to joggers who have been reported in the press as having sustained sudden heart attacks — even died — while engaging in their favorite sport.

The truth is that heart attacks during exercise do not seem to occur in healthy people. Ernst Jokl, M.D., professor of sports medicine at the University of Louisville School of Medicine Health Sciences Center reviewed more than eighty cases of sudden death during exercise, and found that literally all occurred in people with abnormal hearts or blood vessels.

Barry Maron, M.D. of the National Heart, Lung and Blood Institute has presented the same findings.

It's true that exercise could possibly harm a sick heart. Gabe Mirkin, M.D. described how it happens: The blood supply to the heart comes from coronary arteries in its outer surface. The blood on its way to the lungs which is pumped inside the heart carries almost no oxygen. During exercise, the heart works harder and faster to send increased amounts of blood throughout the body. Thus, to meet the increased need for oxygen, the heart requires far more blood to pass through the surface blood vessels. If they are narrowed so that blood supply cannot be increased, the heart muscle can suffer from an oxygen deficiency.

When an oxygen deficit happens, the normal electrical impulses that start the heart beating in a regular and rhythmic fashion are disrupted, and the heart can beat so irregularly that eventually it may not be able to pump blood through the body.

For a person to die while exercising, his heart must be deprived of its blood supply and develop an irregular beat, or he must rupture a blood vessel somewhere in his body. This is the circumstance for those studied by Drs. Jokl and Maron. The victims of heart attack did not have healthy hearts to begin with, and they overtaxed themselves by supplying inadequate quantities of nourishing blood to their damaged hearts and blood vessels.[7]

Rebounding provides a quick and easy aerobic effect to the body, especially the heart. Rebounding could practically be described as a "heart exercise," since in using the rebound exercise unit your legs are the primary limbs physically active. It is easier on the heart to exercise the legs than the arms. Your heart has to work 250 percent harder to pump the same amount of blood through your arms as it does to pump it through your legs. This is why people die while shoveling snow in wintertime. It is not due to the cold weather. Their arm movements are placing a tremendous burden on the heart muscle to deliver oxygen and nutrients in the blood to the upper limbs. When people with weak hearts shovel snow, they can develop heart attacks.

In summary, perform the heart efficiency measurement we described earlier to determine how well you are in shape. First, exercise well on the rebounding de-

---

[7]Gabe Mirkin. "Death on the run." *The Runner* (December 1979), p. 11.

vice to acquire an aerobic effect. Immediately after stopping, check your pulse by placing your fingers on the side of your neck at the carotid artery. Count your pulse. Get the number of beats per minute. In sixty seconds, take a pulse count again. If your pulse rate does not slow down at least twenty-five beats a minute in the first minute after you stop rebounding, you may be in poor shape.

If you have a resting heart rate of less than sixty beats a minute, don't smoke, keep your cholesterol blood level low, don't have chest pain, live a healthful lifestyle, and engage in rebounding aerobics for forty minutes or more per day at least five days out of every week, it's not likely you'll ever develop a heart problem if you have none now.

3

Exercising for One's Life

Forty-nine year-old Ed Pelegrini is a foot doctor and former colleague of medical journalist Morton Walker, D.P.M. Dr. Pelegrini has a certain scholarly charm projected by his receding hair line, acknowledged podiatric skill, and perpetually cheerful grin. The foot-sore patients who visit him for treatment in Lakewood, a suburb of Denver, are grateful to have him doing his utmost to assist their ills — and his own. Dr. Pelegrini has a mesothelioma, a malignant cancer of the pleural lining of the lung, the type suffered by now deceased movie star Steve McQueen.

In 1978, the podiatrist experienced chronic pain in the upper right quadrant of his back. His visit to different orthopedists netted the opinion that he was suffering from an occupational back strain. In podiatry, the professional must bend over a great deal to examine ankles, heels, and toes and to treat corns, callouses, and toenails.

Despite the application of various comforting modalities, the patient's back pain did not improve. Eventually, Dr. Pelegrini found himself forced to give up the various recreational activities he engaged in such as frequent golfing and jogging and to limit practice of his profession.

Finally the man traveled to the Mayo Clinic in Rochester, Minnesota, where a chest surgeon found fluid over his right lung. Exploratory surgery was carried out, observations made, and the surgeon came to the shocking conclusion that without radiation therapy, this new cancer victim could expect to live only six more months. Worse, even with standard chemotherapy or radiation, it was likely he would be dead inside of a year.

Dr. Pelegrini did go through anti-cancer radiation, which accomplished little to stop the progress of his disease. It looked like he was doomed, and he went about putting his affairs in order and preparing his family for what must be inevitable. Yet, he couldn't bring himself to give up the fight, so the patient investigated on his own to seek alternative cancer therapies.

He went to Indianapolis to participate in an experimental procedure consisting of hyperthermia, a treatment involving the heating of the body slightly higher than 106° F for a prolonged period. This overheating is predicated on the fact that cancer cells are more sensitive to heat than normal cells. In some cases, the cancer dies.

Dr. Pelegrini was one of the lucky ones to have his body respond well to the heat treatments. His lung involvement came under control, and he returned home determined to do everything else possible to help himself.

In Denver, The Presbyterian Medical Center had founded its Cancer Self-Help Program in 1976, which supplements conventional medical treatments for cancer with psychological counseling, biofeedback, stress control, mood control, and — most important — exercise. Upon entering the program, Dr. Pelegrini was given an exercise stress test and told he could train with moderation, even though he had only about 40 percent capacity in his right lung.

The cancer victim's new exercise schedule was exhausting and painful; he couldn't walk even for half a block. Still, he reached into himself and found the will to continue trying to rid his body of cancer. He wanted to live.

Gradually the man worked up to an exercise routine of thirty minutes every other day. The more he moved, the more the muscles of his chest expanded and his pain diminished. "One of the mistakes people [cancer patients] make is waiting until they feel better to exercise," he said. "So they stay still and the pain never goes away. If you have a disease like cancer and strong treatments on top of that, you have to rise above it somehow and force yourself to be active."

As this podiatrist exercises, he imagines his body getting stronger and fighting off the remaining disease. "When I'm starting to breathe heavily, I feel that I'm bringing in gobs of oxygen to reinforce the good cells and help them destroy the bad ones," he explained. (As you'll see later in this chaper, Dr. Pelegrini is actually accomplishing what he envisions.)

Although his cough and some pain do return from time to time, exercise has changed the quality of life for Ed Pelegrini. For him, being active means being well. "I feel 100 times better than when I was diagnosed," he said with his perpetual grin. "A year ago, I'd come home with pain and I couldn't do anything. Now I don't have pain, and my lung capacity is twice what it was. It's made me an evangelist with cancer patients who don't want to get up and do anything."[1]

What Exercise Does to Prevent Cancer

Nutritionist Nathan Pritikin, famous for his diet and exercise program, was director of two California institutions: the Longevity Research Institute of Santa Barbara and the Longevity Center of Santa Monica. We

---

[1]Jonathan B. Tucker. "Running for their lives." *The Runner*, (June 1980), 72-76.

listened to his lecture on cancer and how he described it as not being a single disease. "There might be one hundred kinds of cancers," Pritikin said. "The principle types which kill us are lung cancer, number one, probably affecting 70,000 Americans a year. Then there is colon cancer, causing 40,000 deaths a year. Breast cancer is the leading cause of death for women thirty-five to fifty-five years of age. Overall, three hundred thousand lives are lost to cancer each year or at least 16 percent of everyone who dies annually in this country. It used to be thought cancer was caused by viruses, and because of that our government has spent for research probably $100 million a year for twenty years looking for the virus that causes these cancers. They have never found this virus. And now we know they may never find it."

Pritikin blamed the unnatural lifestyle practices by our population as the chief reason for the variety of cancers affecting us. He noted that the sedentary way of life inherent in our white collar occupations and our usual spectator sport leisure pastimes provide insufficient oxygenation of a person's cells. Body cells have to struggle for their full complement of life-giving oxygen molecules, and they break down as a result.

Pritikin used colon cancer as an example: Certain anaerobic type of bacteria grow in the last four feet of tubing comprising one's large intestine. Anaerobic bacteria live without oxygen. They are nasty, because when they eat the bile that comes out of your intestinal tract they convert their excretion products to a cancer-producing substance called **deoxycholic acid.** They also convert their wastes to estrogens (female hormones).

Denis Burkitt, M.D., the noted British internist who first identified and described a certain malignancy found in African children, now known as **Burkitt's lymphoma,** states that the deoxycholic acid and anaerobic excretion products are lodged exactly at the site where colon cancer forms. With regular exercise, quantities of oxygen are carried in the blood stream to the colon. These anaerobic bacteria cannot live in such an unfavorable atmosphere. Oxygen is poison to them. Instead, a different type of bacteria (aerobic) that thrive on oxygen develop in the colon. They are unable to manufacture deoxycholic acid from bile and don't excrete estrogen end products. Therefore, colon cancer is rarely found in actively exercising individuals because of the oxygenation of their colon cells.

Lung cancer may be initiated by cigarette smoking, asbestos dust, or the inhalation of other toxic powders or pollutants. In the case of podiatrist Ed Pelegrini, he might have brought on his lung involvement by inhaling the nail dust he created from grinding patients' toenails during the course of his work.

The newest finding by exercise physiologists is that oxygenation of the lung tissues from taking in large quantities of fresh air while exercising tends to lower the incidence of lung cancer.

Not only this, but Pritikin cited Jeremiah Stamler, M.D., of Chicago's Board of Health, who conducted studies on lung cancer. Ten years ago Dr. Stamler tested 900 people for a relationship between the number of cigarettes they smoked and lung cancer. He couldn't tie the relationship together, but he did find a connection between their elevated blood cholesterol levels and lung cancer. If the subjects' serum cholesterol level was 275 milligrams percent (mg %), or more, there was eight times as many cases of lung cancer than if the serum cholesterol was 220 mg %, or less. Of the people checked having serum cholesterol levels below 150 mg %, there wasn't any lung cancer present among this group.

Why does this anti-cancer, low-cholesterol effect occur? It's because high cholesterol blood paralyzes the action of white blood cells that eat cancer cells. The macrophage, a white blood cell fifty times larger than an ordinary red blood cell, travels through the tissues looking for foreign substances to eat. When it comes upon a cancer cell, the macrophage attacks it and digests it. But blood with an elevated cholesterol level removes the mobility from the millions of macrophages traveling in the blood and prevents their immune reaction from taking place. Cancer cells lodged in the lung (cancer cells are in the body at all times) will likely be allowed to multiply when macrophages are prevented from making their attack. And a high blood cholesterol level is a main cause.

Vigorous aerobic exercise causes a reduction in blood pressure, especially in individuals with hypertension, as we stated in chapter two. Additionally, the chemistry of the blood is modified. The blood contains two principal classes of fats: cholesterol and the lesser-known triglycerides. The level of both substances in the blood is influenced by many factors, the most important of which are diet and exercise. Everybody has heard that excessive cholesterol increases the probability of heart attack, but less than a year ago medical scientists learned about too much cholesterol protecting cancer cells from being attacked by white blood cells.

Thus, exercise is known to affect both cholesterol and triglycerides: often dramatically lowering both of them, especially in people who have relatively high levels to begin with.

Moreover, recent research has shown that the total level of cholesterol in the blood is not as important as the ratio of high-density to low-density lipoproteins, the protein compounds that transport the cholesterol. Low-density lipoproteins (LDL) are the villains. They carry cholesterol into the tissues and thicken the blood. High-density lipoproteins (HDL), on the other hand, have the opposite effect. "High-density is the body's sewer system," says Dr. Arthur S. Leon of the University of Minnesota Medical School, in an interview. "The only way the body has to get rid of cholesterol from the arteries and other tissues is this carrier protein that carries it to the liver, which can degrade it and throw it out."

In proving that HDL stimulated by aerobic exercise

protects a person against cancer, heart disease, and other degenerative diseases, a study was conducted at Methodist Hospital in Houston and published in the February 14, 1980 issue of the *New England Journal of Medicine*. The study found the more people engaged in aerobic exercises such as rebounding, running, bicycling, swimming, rope skipping, and similar activities, the higher their blood levels of HDL.

The researchers said it was the amount of exercise, not what people ate, that determined whether they had high or low levels of this blood fat. Among the subjects tested, all men, 144 were very active or moderately active exercisers and 74 were inactive. HDL levels were 65 mg per deciliter of blood in the very active, 58 mg in the moderately active, and 43 mg in the non-active. "The exercisers did not differ substantially from the inactive subjects in their reported dietary habits, although they had significantly higher HDL-cholesterol levels," the researchers wrote. They attributed the differences to the men's exercising habits.[2]

Aerobic exercise of various types and mental relaxation utilizing several techniques are all employed by the Cancer Self-Help Program of the Denver Presbyterian Medical Center. According to Paul K. Hamilton, M.D., a medical oncologist in Denver, about half of all cancer patients receiving therapy are capable of and should engage in mild exercise. Unfortunately, he finds that only a small percentage of cancer patients are willing to exercise, even while they show no signs of the disease being present. They think of themselves as fragile human beings ready to shatter at any exertion even though the only time there really is such fragility is when a tumor spreads to the bones and makes a person more susceptible to spontaneous fracture.

Rebounding aerobics and other forms of aerobic exercise provide many emotionally lifting effects for a

---

[2]Daniel Q. Honey. "Researchers link running to heart disease reduction." *The Advocate*. February 14, 1980, p. 55.

cancer patient, too. T. Flint Sparks, the director of counseling for the Cancer Self-Help Program, said that anti-cancer aerobics is beneficial both psychologically and physiologically. The psychological lift includes a greater feeling of control over one's life, an improved self-image, and reduced depression.

"All our patients are self-selected and unrepresentative of the general cancer-patient population in that they've been willing to participate in their own treatment," said Sparks. "One thing that characterizes our patients is the need to take charge of their lives and not follow the crowd. In oncology, following the crowd usually means dying."

Cellular Abnormalities Can Be Prevented with Exercise

A fearless — and peppery — champion of truth, Otto Heinrich Warburg, M.D., is the most distinguished of a generation of great German biochemists. In 1931, Dr. Warburg received the Nobel Prize in physiology and medicine for his identification of the oxygen-activating respiratory enzyme as an iron porphyrin derivative. His main scientific interests centered around three fundamental biological phenomena: cellular respiration, photosynthesis, and cancer. The impact of his contributions in all of these areas is difficult to overestimate.

Dr. Warburg says that carcinogens such as food additives, smoking, air pollution, soil pollution, water pollution, and other things blamed as the causes of cancer are not the true villains. They are only the circumstances that set the scene for cellular abnormalities to take place. But the real cause that stimulates a single cell to start subdividing spontaneously, quickly, and without any discernible pattern to its mitosis is the lack of oxygen at the cellular level.

As we have implied in the previous paragraphs, oxygen starvation causes cells to turn from respiration to fermentation in order to obtain their energy. Whereas normally the cells obtain their energy, life force, multiplication stimulus, exchange of waste products for nutrition, and other functions of life in the presence of oxygen, pathological cells that turn cancerous go through another process. They break down glucose and other sugars without the use of oxygen. They ferment into the condition known as cancer.

Cancer cells survive and grow fat in an oxygen-free environment, and the only other cells in nature with such anaerobic properties are particular fungi. At the level of the cell, anaerobic conditions favorable for the growth of cancer will have normal cells die and abnormal cells with the potential for harmful change thrive. This circumstance surely will be true if the body's natural defenses are down.

The person who does not exercise has a lowered defense system. Ordinary breathing often takes in an overabundant quantity of polluted air, especially if you live in an industrialized environment. Intermixed among gases of industrialization are carbon dioxide and carbon monoxide. You get no oxygen nutrition from carbon dioxide and suffer the stealing of oxygen molecules by carbon monoxide. Polluted air actually robs any oxygen stored in your body by forcing it to combine chemically with carbon monoxide molecules you take in from the air.

Your not exercising fails to give any stimulus to your blood to circulate and no pumping from the muscles takes place. The capillaries tend to constrict and rather than nourishing the peripheral parts of the body such as the skin and limbs, they carry the blood inward merely to nourish the vital organs. The body retains little of its resources to fight off assaults from toxic heavy metals, poisonous chemicals, some foreign proteins or invasion by unfriendly viruses or bacteria.

Lack of exercise provides no abundance of oxygen to the cells to help them defend against disease. Deoxygenation of cells is a prime cause of cancer at the cellular level. In his 1966 address before the Nobel Committee upon accepting his second Nobel Prize, Dr. Warburg said:

> The great advantage of knowing the prime cause of a disease is that it can then be attacked logically and over a broad front. This is particularly important in the case of cancer, with its numerous secondary and remote causes, and because it is often stated that in man alone there are over one hundred well-known and quite different kinds of cancer, usually with the implication that therefore we will have to find one or several hundred bases for prevention and treatment, and usually without any realization that this need not necessarily be the case now that we know that all cancers studied have a characteristic metabolism in common, a prime cause.[3]

Being informed that the prime cause of cancer is lack of oxygenation of the cells, and knowing well that exercise is the main way to bring oxygen into the blood with which to bathe the cells, it's logical to adopt routine exercising as part of your daily lifestyle. Isn't it?

Breast Cancer Changes from Estrogen

Nathan Pritikin had pointed out that not only do the anaerobic bacteria produce the carcinogen deoxycholic acid, but also they convert their waste products to estrogens. The estrogens are reabsorbed back into a woman's body and bring on a variety of cancer-like changes.

Pritikin told the story of a three-and-a-half year old girl who secretly applied her mother's estrogen face cream all over her body for a couple of months. Her mother discovered the little girl was doing this by observing the child's breasts beginning to grow. Then, examination by a pediatrician uncovered that the youngster's uterus resembled a normal, adult, menstruating female organ. From smearing her skin with cream, the

---

[3]"The Prime Cause and Prevention of Cancer," revised lecture of the Nobel-Laureates on June 30, 1966 at Lindau, Lake Constance, Germany by Otto Warburg, translated by Dean Burk. (Dean Burk was a close research associate with Otto Warburg during the time they studied the energetics of photosynthesis.)

little girl had absorbed only one-twentieth of the amount of estrogen to bring on such changes and yet, she showed characteristics of being a mature woman. This shows how potent estrogen can be.

Indeed, planned parenthood statistics indicate that women taking oral contraceptives and other estrogen products tend to develop cysts in the uterus within six months. The national Planned Parenthood League studied groups of women who were perfectly healthy and free of fibrous cysts in the uterus. An examination of these women six months after they started on estrogen oral contraceptives revealed that 25 percent of them had grown uterine cysts. After two years on the estrogen pills, 80 percent developed such cysts. Gynecologists have proven that the presence of uterine cysts increases a woman's risk of breast cancer by 260 percent.

Women who took the estrogen hormone diethylstilbestrol (DES) for controlling miscarriage have been followed closely and been found to increase their rate of cancer over those who did not take DES.

Premarine is the estrogen taken by some women to stay young-looking. Ingesting premarine tablets for two years has been shown to elevate a woman's chance of getting cancer of the uterus by 400 percent. If premarine is ingested regularly for seven years or more, the uterine cancer risk jumps fourteen to one, a 1400 percent greater incidence for a woman than if she did not take the youth drug.

Estrogens are a known potent force in the development of female body changes. Why are today's girls age ten, eleven, and twelve experiencing their first menstruation prematurely when for hundreds of thousands of years during the evolution of the human race, menstruation had not appeared until young women reached ages sixteen, seventeen, and eighteen? This is occurring because during the past fifty or one hundred years, women in highly industrialized western countries find it unnecessary to move around to perform their daily chores as they had in prior times. They have labor-saving devices which take away the need to exercise in accomplishing necessary work. From childhood on they have colonies of anaerobic bacteria in their bodies building up quantities of estrogen, because of their lessened activity.

We are now beginning to realize that labor-saving devices are not necessarily life-saving. The insufficient exercise that goes along with high technology allows for too much anaerobic bacteria growth in a woman's bowel, lungs, breasts, uterus, ovaries, and other organs. The anaerobes produce unnatural estrogens which are toxic, carcinogenic, and disease-producing. The result is an alarming jump in annual death statistics from breast, cervical, ovarian, and uterine cancers in the in-dustrialized western countries, especially among women in the United States.

Any woman who has the knowledge and motivation can exercise herself away from cancer. Susan Russell of Boulder, Colorado, age thirty-four, is doing this now, except it's after she has already come down with breast cancer. She became frightened and confused in 1977 after she learned of her deadly disease. "I didn't know what would happen to me," she said. "My daughter was two at the time, and I worried a lot about her not having a mother."

Following a radical mastectomy and five weeks of radiation therapy at M.D. Anderson Hospital in Houston, Mrs. Russell began a concentrated program of aerobic exercises. "I feel my blood surging, and I think of the image of the healthy body I'm striving toward," she said. "I used to worry a lot about the pos-sibility of a recurrence, but now I feel I'm doing one more thing to make sure the cancer doesn't come back."[4]

Might it not be wise for women to make exercise a part of their lifestyles before cancer strikes?

---

[4]Tucker, *Op. cit. p.* 73.

What's the Best Anti-Cancer Exercise?

What about the current convictions held by Ed Pelegrini and Susan Russell? Certainly it's likely they wish they had engaged in an anti-cancer exercise program before becoming victims of the dread disease. Regular daily physical activity is something you could engage in as a method of prevention or for therapeutic purposes in the event that cancer has become part of your involvement with living.

All exercise is not alike, however. Some is good for your muscles by improving their strength. Other exercise promotes skills, and may improve your tennis stroke or paddleball game, but won't make you stronger. Still other kinds of exercise may challenge your cardiovascular system, enhancing your endurance, wind, and the oxygenation of your blood. The latter is the form of activity that may be considered a preventive or therapeutic measure against cancer. It should be long in duration, moderate in intensity, administered daily, and performed for a lifetime. The exercise you choose may become part of your lifestyle, because it's easy and fun and the gain in tissue oxygenation increases as the duration of exercise increases. During the time you are taking it, the exercise should be rhythmic, repetitive and continuous, to promote the intake of air, a steady flow of blood, and full nourishment to body tissues.

Although weight loss from exercising often does occur, losing pounds is not our main goal here. Weight control is just a fringe benefit. You'd have to run vigorously for fifteen minutes to burn off the calories of a single eclair, bicycle rapidly for thirteen minutes for a baked potato without butter, or swim nine minutes for the number of calories eaten in a single apple. Any weight loss bonus comes in from exercising at a moderate level, done regularly over a long period. It can also help you maintain your goal weight if daily exercise becomes a habit and is an activity which you enjoy, find convenient, and want to continue. You don't have to run yourself ragged, or end up with a sprain or a strain. Moderate-level, long-duration, lifetime exercise can effectively and permanently keep your body's tissues filled with the oxygen you seek as a protective component against degenerative disease like cancer.

Lenore R. Zohman, M.D., a specialist in the field of cardiopulmonary rehabilitation, developed a fitness point system for Weight Watchers International, Inc., which the company incorporated into their clients' personal exercise plan and called "Pepstep." We have been given permission to use Dr. Zohman's system of *Strenuous Points* shown in Tables II, III, and IV so that you may adapt it as your own technique for finding how physically fit you are. Learning of the extent of your fitness, you'll possibly be able to discover what is the best anti-cancer exercise for you.

Table II

Instructions

Think of the most strenuous activity (activities) you do and determine your point score by comparing your strenuous physical activities with the description below. Write your "Strenuousness Points" in the scoring formula.

Points	Strenuousness Points
5	**Very Heavy** - Continuous heavy effort resulting in rapid heart action or heavy breathing as long as you keep up this activity — like running, fast cycling, competitive handball. You burn approximately 10-12 calories per minute.
4	**Heavy** - Bursts of effort which cause rapid heart action or heavy breathing — like vigorous singles tennis, downhill skiing, basketball, folk dancing; 8-10 calories per minute.
3	**Moderate** - Requires moderate extra effort and works up a sweat — like very fast walking, jogging, playing a sport, cycling, skating; 6-8 calories per minute.
2	**Light** - Requires very little extra effort and is usually intermittent — like volleyball, ping-pong, playing catch, golf with a cart, mopping and scrubbing floors; 4-6 calories per minute.
1	**Minimal** — Involves customary level of effort — like strolling or a short walk, most other household activities; 2-4 calories per minute.

Table III

Points	Time Period
5	30 minutes or more
4	20-29 minutes
3	10-19 minutes
2	5-9 minutes
1	less than 5 minutes

Time Points

Now think about how much time you spend doing that most strenuous activity. That is, each time you do that activity how long do you keep at it? Find your points for time spent. Write your time period in the scoring formula.

Points	Regularity
5	daily
4	3-6 times/week
3	1-2 times/week
2	1-3 times/month
1	less than 1 time/month

Regularity Points

Think about how often you do that strenuous activity in a day, a week, or a month. Enter your regularity score in the scoring formula.

Scoring Formula*

$$\text{Strenuousness Points} \times \text{Time Points} \times \text{Regularity Points} = \text{Your Fitness Score is:}$$

$$\times \quad\quad \times \quad\quad =$$

*Multiply **Strenuousness Points** times **Time Points** times **Regularity Points** to determine your Fitness Score.

Table IV
Interpretation

Fitness Score	Fitness Level	Significance
100	Excellent	You are in great shape. Maintain this activity level.
60-99	Good	You are in good shape and should maintain at least the activity you do now.
40-59	Average	At least you aren't sedentary, but you could be more active.
20-39	Below Average	You are moderately sedentary and should be more active.
Less than 20	Poor	You need exercise most of all!

My Fitness Level is _____

According to Robert E. Johnson, M.D., Ph.D. of the University of Illinois College of Medicine, a 150-pound person will burn the following number of calories per hour (cph) while participating in an activity:

Activity	cph
Lying down or sleeping	80
Sitting	100
Driving a car	120
Standing	140
Domestic work	180
Walking 2.5 mph	210
Bicycling 5.5 mph	210
Gardening	220
Golfing	250
Lawn mowing with power mower	250
Bowling	270
Walking 3.75 mph	300
Swimming 1/4 mile	300
Square dancing	350
Volleyball playing	350
Roller skating	350
Wood chopping or sawing	400
Tennis playing	420
Cross country skiing 10 mph	600
Squash playing	600
Handball playing	600
Bicycling 13 mph	660
Running 10 mph	900

Clearly, burning 3,500 calories which would have your lose about one pound of bulk from your body is not that easy to do. This accounts for the fact that many studies have shown little difference between obese and thin people as regards their activity levels. The number of calories associated with various activities are instructive nonetheless, since you're able to see which tend toward being aerobic in their effects.

There are millions of people who have been serious runners for years, but who cannot cover ten miles in an hour. On the other hand, there are plenty of golfers who claim they are getting ample exercise playing eighteen holes.

To unravel the confusion about which is the best anti-cancer exercise because it infuses excellent increments of oxygen into the body for the number of calories of energy expended, we have furnished **Table V.**[5] In this table, energy expenditure is expressed in three ways: (1) in multiples of "metabolic units" called **mets,** which are the basal oxygen requirements of your body at rest and are equivalent to 3/5 milliliters of oxygen per minute per kilogram. (ml O_2/min/kg) of body weight, (2) in terms of actual oxygen consumption, and (3) in terms of calories expended per minute (cal/min). Exercise equivalents provided in the table are also in three categories: (a) exercise, (b) work, and (c) play.

Table V

Energy Levels		Exercise Equivalents	
(1)	1½ - 2 mets	(a)	Standing, walking at 1 mph, operating a car under ordinary stress conditions.
	or		
(2)	4 - 7 ml O_2/min/kg	(b)	Ordinary desk work, operating an electric office machine, sewing, knitting
	or		
(3)	2 - 2½ cal/min	(c)	Playing cards

[5]Adapted from S.M. Fox; J.P. Naughton; and P.A. Gorman. "Physical activity and cardiovascular health (Table V), *Modern Concepts of Cardiovascular Disease.* Volume 41, Number 6, pp. 27 and 28.

Energy Levels	**Exercise Equivalents**
(1) 2 - 3 mets or (2) 7 - 11 ml O₂ min/kg or (3) 2½ - 4 cal/min	(a) Level walking (2 mph), level bicycling (5 mph) (b) Manual typewriting, auto or radio-TV repair, light janitorial work, bartending, riding a lawn mower (c) Playing billiards, shuffle-board, or piano, bowling, skeet-shooting, light woodworking, powerboat driving, playing golf (with power cart), horseback riding at a walk, canoeing at 2½ mph
(1) 3 - 4 mets or (2) 11 - 14 ml O₂/min/kg or (3) 4 - 5 cal/min	(a) Walking at 3 mph, cycling at 6 mph (b) Machine assembly-line work, driving a trailer truck in traffic, moderate welding, window cleaning, brick-laying, plastering, pushing a small power mower or light wheelbarrow load (c) Horseshoe pitching, six-man non-competitive volleyball, playing golf (pulling a bag cart), archery, sailing a small boat, fly fishing at a stand, non-competitive badminton (doubles)
(1) 4 -5 mets or (2) 14 - 18 ml O₂/min/kg or (3) 5 - 6 cal/min	(a) Walking at 3½ mph, cycling at 8 mph (b) Painting, paperhanging, light carpentry, raking leaves, hoeing (c) Table tennis, playing golf (carrying clubs), badminton (singles), or tennis (doubles)

Energy Levels	Exercise Equivalents
(1) 5 - 6 mets or (2) 18 - 21 ml O_2/min/kg or (3) 6 - 7 cal/min	(a) Walking at 4 mph, cycling at 10 mph (b) Digging a garden, light dirt shoveling (c) Ice or roller skating at 9 mph, fishing against a light current, canoeing at 4 mph, horseback riding at a trot
(1) 6 - 7 mets or (2) 21 - 25 ml O_2/min/kg or (3) 7 - 8 cal/min	(a) Walking at 5 mph, cycling at 11 mph (b) Shoveling dirt at the rate of ten 10-lb. loads/min, pushing a hand mower, splitting wood, snow shoveling (c) Playing competitive badminton or tennis (singles), folk dancing, light downhill skiing, cross-country skiing at 2½ mph in loose snow, water skiing
(1) 7 - 8 mets or (2) 25 - 28 ml O_2/min/kg or (3) 8 - 10 cal/min	(a) Jogging at 5 mph, cycling at 12 mph (b) Sawing hardwood, digging ditches, carrying an 80-lb. work load (c) Horseback riding at a gallop, vigorous downhill skiing, playing basketball, ice hockey, touch football, or paddleball, canoeing at 5 pmh, mountain climbing
(1) 8 - 9 mets or (2) 28 - 32 ml O_2/min/kg or (3) 10 - 11 cal/min	(a) Running at 5½ mph, cycling at 13 mph (b) Shoveling dirt (ten 14-lb. loads/min) (c) Playing noncompetitive squash or handball, vigorous basketball, fencing, cross-country skiing at 4 mph in loose snow

Energy Levels		Exercise Equivalents	
(1)	10 mets	(a)	Running at 6 mph
	or		
(2)	32 ml O_2/min/kg	(b)	Shoveling dirt (ten 16-lb loads/min)
	or		
(3)	11 cal/min	(c)	Competitive handball or squash, cross-country skiing at 5 mph

Your rate of rebounding will vary with the amount of effort you put into the bounce and the height you lift your feet from the mat to speed up or slow down the bounce. Therefore, rebounding will give you the ideal aerobic effect with almost any rate of performance, because it fills all the requisites of an oxygenating exercise. Rebounding lets you prolong its duration, increase or decrease its intensity, engage in it regularly, employ it for a lifetime, and adjust it to your level of fitness. Of all the exercise activities available to mankind, rebounding aerobics becomes the perfect physical movement. It is more beneficial physiologically, therapeutically, and for its protective effects against degenerative diseases, especially cancer, than any other form of motion in the workplace, in recreational pursuits, or in exercising simply for the care of your body.

Your ability to vary rebounding aerobics and tailor them to your personal needs at the time you are filling those needs is what puts these series of movements into a state of complete excellence. They provide you with the best available cellular oxidation for counteracting invading carcinogens.

4

Lymphatic Cleansing from Instant Aerobics

A thirteen-year-old girl living in Parkersburg, West Virginia, whom we'll call Cathy B. to protect her identity, suffered from chronic swelling of her left leg. It had begun during the end of her eleventh year, developing slowly but steadily getting worse. The leg was now twice the diameter of her right, especially at the ankle and just below the knee.

The swelling did not hurt, and examination by several physicians could find no discernable cause. She finally was diagnosed as suffering from **primary idiopathic lymphedema,** also known as **lymphedema praecox.** This medical terminology simply meant that Cathy had a disorder affecting the lymphatic system from no known cause, appearing insidiously and prematurely. First it had taken the form of some puffiness about the ankle which then spread upward onto the leg, eventually involving the entire limb. At the onset, the degree of swelling appeared to be increased by such factors as standing, sitting, and hot weather. When she began her menstrual cycle at age twelve, the girl then experienced a ballooning of her left leg just before the start of her menses. Even without feeling any cramps, Cathy and her mother could predict each month that menstruation would be starting for her in a few days merely from observing the increased size of the teen's one leg.

There was nothing much to be done, her doctors said. Bed rest did relieve the swelling, and usually it would entirely disappear after a night's sleep. But staying in bed was not a way of life for an active and budding young lady. Besides, the accumulation of fluid during the day became progessively greater, while the effect of recumbency on reducing it was less and less marked.

By the time Cathy turned fourteen, her leg became susceptible to attacks of acute lymphangitis, which is an inflammation of the lymphatic channels, usually caused by streptococcus or staphylococcus bacteria. During one of those attacks she often felt morose, depressed, achy all over, had severe headaches, chills, and was in danger of having the infection spread. It was necessary for her to take large doses of antibiotics.

Seemingly, she was doomed to go through life with one oversized leg, and this had her frantic anytime a social occasion arose. Few boys would date her. No remedy helped Cathy's condition, and the girl wished someone would accede to her demand when she said, "Cut off my leg!"

By chance, Cathy's father bought himself a rebounding device to use at his place of business, an insurance office. He knew that he failed to get enough exercise working at his sedentary occupation. However, the man's boss frowned on any activity which took one of the workers away from selling insurance and servicing clients. Cathy's father, consequently, was forced to bring home his rebound unit and leave it to gather dust in a corner.

The teenager discovered this device that she considered a toy — a fun thing — which she danced on to music in the privacy of her room. As it was, the girl avoided companions from feeling so self-conscious about her big ugly leg. For hours at a time, days on end, she jogged and jumped on the rebound device using different steps to the beat, beat, beat of her rock-and-roll records.

She first noticed that her leg wasn't swelling any-more when for the second month in succession, right on schedule, her menstruation came without any prior warning. Her usually larger left leg just did not swell enough to let the girl know that the menstrual flow would start in a few days. Its arrival came as a surprise.

Cathy alerted her mother, and together they watched for her next month's period, keeping an eye on the size of her leg as the usual method of prediction. But the leg did not swell anymore. The appearance of her menses was like any normal young woman's with no particular announcement of its arrival. If anything, it was milder and she felt less crampy than ever.

About this time, Cathy went on an out-of-town trip to visit her invalid grandmother for three weeks. She left behind her favorite exercising device. In fact, the young woman hardly did any exercise, since her grandmother's wish was for Cathy to sit with her a lot and carry on long conversations.

When her menstrual period appeared the following month it was preceded by moderate swelling of her left leg. The lymphedema had returned but not as severely as it had been. Cathy and her mother deduced that the rebounding exercises the girl habitually engaged in were the relief-giving remedy that was bringing about the end of her misery.

It's more than a year now that Cathy's case history came to our attention. Her leg swelling doesn't return, she tells us, as long as she continues her program of re-bounding aerobics. It's an activity this pretty young woman performs faithfully, you can be sure.

The Lymphatic Drainage System

Aerobic movement provides the stimulus for a free-flowing lymphatic drainage system. The lymphatic system is the metabolic garbage can of the body. It rids the body of toxins, fatigue substances, dead cells, cancer cells, nitrogenous wastes, trapped protein, fatty globules, pathogenic bacteria, infectious viruses, foreign substances, heavy metals, and other assorted junk the cells cast off. Removal of these components derived from metabolic breakdown (catabolism) takes away potential poisonings anyone is better off without.

Young Cathy B. had been the victim of a malfunctioning lymphatic system. For a reason unknown to her doctors, the young woman had undergone a spontaneous blockage of the involved lymph channels. Persistent lymphedema and numerous inflammatory episodes, resulted in stagnation of lymphatic fluid flow. This produced thickening of the walls of her formerly open lymph vessels and hence accentuation of the process. It was a vicious cycle which might eventually have placed the girl's life in danger if Cathy had not accidentally discovered her own way out of the condition.[1]

The lymphatic drainage system is a highly complex portion of the body's cardiovascular circulatory tree. In this chapter, we will endeavor to explain how it works without using too much technical detail.

After the systemic circulatory system conveys food and oxygen to living cells by means of nutritional transfer from the blood, the products of catabolism must eventually be drained away with its load of wastes through the lymphatic ducts. There is a never-ending problem with lymphatic circulation (and to a lesser extent with venous circulation). Unlike the arterial system, the lymphatics do not have their own pump. There are just three ways to activate and speed up the flow of

---

[1]F.P. Chinard. "Starling's hypothesis in the formation of edema." *Bulletin of the N.Y. Acad. Med.* 38 (1962) p. 375.

lymph away from the tissues it serves and back into the main pulmonary circulation. Lymphatic flow requires:

1. Muscular contraction from exercise and movement.
2. Gravitational pressure.
3. Internal massage to the valves of the lymph ducts.

Rebound exercise does supply all three for anybody interested in moving waste products out of the cells and out of the body. Cellular cleansing takes place quite well from this instant aerobic movement.

If an individual is inactive for a long time, the lymph will not flow nearly enough to flush away normal waste substances from his cells. A varying level of toxicity will exist throughout much of the body. This is why, for example, a perfectly healthy person confined to bed for an extended period because of a broken leg will end up feeling just plain terrible. His own toxins will have accumulated to poison the cells in his vital organs.

Aside from poor nutrition, the primary cause of fatigue, disease, cell degeneration, and resultant premature aging is poor circulation to and from the tissues of the body. There is resultant stagnation of cellular fluids. Living cells and organs, when continually supplied with proper nutrients and oxygen, will thrive only so long as toxic waste substances are concurrently removed and regularly excreted from the body. This is the main job of the lymphatic system.

When we effectively move the lymph away from the cells, it becomes easier for arterial blood to enter the capillaries and supply the cells with fresh tissue fluid — food and oxygen. Part of the rationale of rebounding aerobics is that it effectively moves and recycles the lymph and the entire blood supply through the circulatory system many times during the course of the rebounding session. And it begins doing this instantly — even with your first bounce on the rebound unit. Such instant aerobics is the means toward total cellular cleansing.

If the lymphatic ducts get plugged up at their main

junctures to block lymphatic flow, the results would be
fatal. As mentioned, Cathy's condition could have killed
her. Please follow us closely through the next few pages
as we explain how and why good lymphatic functioning
is accomplished so that you may apply the knowledge
for your own benefit.

How Our Cells Rid Themselves of Wastes

More than 75 percent of the body is comprised of
water, primarily in the form of an exceedingly loose protoplasm, called **interstitial fluid.** This interstitial fluid
is the greyish fluid, for example, that oozes out of a
skinned knee when there isn't actually any bleeding of
red cells. A continuous interchange goes on between the
body's trillions of cells and their surrounding interstitial fluids. Food and oxygen are exchanged by the fluids
for waste products from the cells. Arterial pressure
moves the fluid into and out of the cells' interstitial
spaces so that circulation is constantly making this exchange. Fluid filled with toxic waste is picked up by tiny
lymphatic tubules or ducts and sent through the lymph
vessels to be detoxified.

If toxic waste wasn't carried away from the cells in
this way, the living cells would lose their efficiency, or
even die, since their own waste products would act as
poisons. The system of lymphatic ducts taking away the
various toxic components extend everywhere throughout
the body. They resemble the roots of a tree and run
alongside most capillaries, arterioles, and venules.

Be reminded of the exceedingly important fact that
unlike the arterial or venus system, the lymphatic system has no pump in its vessels to push along the lymph
fluid. Instead, lymphatics depend on the contraction
of muscles, passive movement of the parts of the body,
compression of the tissues from the outside, and gravity
to move the fluids filled with waste to their main garbage dumps in the left and right subclavian veins.

At certain spots along the lymphatic channels

spongelike straining stations, called **lymph nodes,** are located to collect toxins of cancerous growths and specific disease-producing bacteria. The nodes prevent the spread of disease by keeping cancer cells localized or infections from infiltrating further. According to immunologist Lawrence Burton, Ph.D., of Nassau, the Bahamas, cancer and infection are always present within our bodies but our natural immunity wards off the effects of these diseases. One of the stimulators of such immunity is exercise.

Arthur C. Guyton, M.D., professor and chairman of the Department of Physiology and Biophysics, University of Mississippi School of Medicine, an internationally famous expert on lymphology, the science of the lymphatic system, says:

> The lymphatic pump becomes very active during exercise but sluggish under resting conditions. During exercise the rate of lymph flow can increase to as high as 3 to 14 times normal because of the increased activity . . . An increase in tissue fluid protein increases the rate of lymph flow, and this washes the proteins out of the tissue spaces, automatically returning the protein concentration to its normal low level. If it were not for this continual removal of proteins, the dynamics of the capillaries would become so abnormal within only a few hours that life could no longer continue. There is certainly no other function of the lymphatics that can even approach this in importance.[2]

Approximately 100 milliliters (ml) of lymph fluid travels to the thoracic duct of a resting person per hour, and perhaps another 20 ml. of lymph flows into the circulation each hour through other channels, making a total estimated lymph fluid flow of 120 ml. per hour. This rate of flow is quite small in comparison with the rate of blood flow.

---

[2]Arthur C. Guyton. *Basic Human Physiology: Normal Function and Mechanisms of Disease.* (Philadelphia: W.B. Saunders Co., 1971), p. 189.

Dr.Guyton tells us that elevation of the interstitial fluid pressure above its normal level of -7 millimeters (mm) of mercury (Hg) increased the flow of interstitial fluid into the lymph vessels at the end of the lymphatic system where they drain the cells of wastes. Increased fluid pressure naturally increases the rate of lymph flow. This increase in flow is relatively even until the interstitial fluid pressure reaches 0, at which point the flow is ten to fifty times normal. Therefore, any factor, besides obstruction of the lymphatic system itself, that tends to increase interstitial fluid pressures increases the rate of lymph flow.

Increased fluid pressure and rate of flow had happened to young Cathy B. It was never discovered which metabolic factor brought on her condition. Her body underwent a spontaneous change evolving from one or more of the following four factors commonly the cause of poor lymphatic system drainage:

1. Elevated capillary pressure (from temporary or permanent hypertension).

2. Decreased plasma colloid osmotic pressure (from inadequate trace minerals in the body).

3. Increased interstitial fluid protein (from a possibly overly abundant intake of animal protein).

4. Increased permeability of the capillaries (from a reaction to alteration of the internal environment).

Moreover, the lymph channels have valves, even down to the tiniest vessels. In the larger lymphatic channels, valves exist every few millimeters, and the smaller lymphatics have valves even closer together than this.

Every time the lymph vessel is compressed by pressure from any source, some lymph tends to be squeezed in both directions, but because the valves are open only in the central direction, the fluid moves just one way, out toward the location of dumping in the thoracic duct and the subclavian junctures.

All the lymph from the lower parts of the body including the legs and torso collects in one major duct (thoracic) that extends along inside the torso to shoulder level where it flows into the left subclavian vein. Lymphatic ducts from the arms, head, and neck also enter the subclavian veins under the collar bones.

Upon flowing this way into the venous blood, the lymph cycles through the lungs, liver, kidneys, and skin to excrete the waste products it carries. And toxins created during the course of ordinary metabolism are sent out of the body.[3]

Certain intrinsic and extrinsic factors affect the pressure of the lymphatics and how effectively they do their job. We had alluded to these factors previously without emphasis. They are:

1. Contraction of muscles (by your own active exercise).

2. Passive movement of the parts of the body (by someone else moving you).

3. Arterial pulsations (by a strong heart beat).

4. Compression of the tissues from the outside (by massage or by the wearing of a non-constrictive corset).

These four circumstances, singularly or collectively, provide a beneficial stimulation to lymphatic flow. The best stimulant is definitely exercise, for the lymphatic pump becomes very efficient during active movement but sluggish under resting conditions. During exercise the rate of lymph flow can increase to as high as three to fourteen times normal because of the increased activity, according to Dr. Guyton. He has devised a formula that determines the rate of lymph flow.[4]

$$\text{the product of tissue pressure} \times \text{the activity of the lymphatic pump} = \text{the rate of lymph flow}$$

---

[3] J.M. Yoffrey and F.C. Courtice. *Lymphatics, Lymph, and Lymphoid Tissue.* Baltimore: The Williams & Wilkins Co., 1967.

[4] A.C. Guyton. "Interstitial fluid pressure-volume relationships and their regulation." In Wolstenholme, G.E.W., and Knight, J. (eds): *Ciba Foundation Symposium on Circulatory and Respiratory Mass Transport.* (London: J. & A. Churchhill Ltd., 1969) p. 4.

The Theory of Trapped Plasma Proteins

Corwin Samuel West, N.D. of Orem, Utah has stated, "I know why people are getting sick, why they are in pain, and why they are degenerating: we have been un-informed about the importance of our lymphatic system — the foundation of health."

Building on Dr. Guyton's investigations and conclusions, West has come up with a simple but reasonable theory for the presence of chronic and acute pain, loss of energy and degenerative disease.

Dr. Guyton pointed out that since blood protein continually leaks from the capillaries into the interstitial fluid spaces, it must also be removed continually. Otherwise the tissue colloid osmotic pressure will become so high that normal capillary dynamics can no longer continue. Sickness and eventual death must follow the blockage of circulation in the spaces around the cells.

By far the most necessary function of the lymphatic system is the maintenance of low protein concentration in the interstitial fluid. As fluid leaks from the arterial ends of the capillaries into the interstitial spaces, only small quantities of protein accompany it. However, as the fluid is reabsorbed into the blood stream to be carried out of the body, most of the protein is left behind.

Dr. Guyton described how the blood protein progressively accumulates in the interstitial fluid, and this in turn increases the tissue colloid osmotic pressure. The osmotic pressure then decreases reabsorption of fluid by the capillaries, thereby promoting increased tissue fluid volume and increased tissue pressure. The increased pressure then forces interstitial fluid into the lymphatic channels, and the fluid carries with it the excess protein that has accumulated. As a result, normal capillary dynamics ensue once again.[5]

However, Dr. West says if you fail to maintain your

---

[5]Arthur C. Guyton. *Textbook of Medical Physiology.* (Philadelphia: W.B. Saunders Co., 1976), pp. 707-985.

level of wellness and let yourself deteriorate, normal capillary dynamics will not resume. Performing your daily tasks in a state of low level wellness, bordering on illness, will cause the lymph channels and capillaries to malfunction.

In lectures, West has said, "The blood protein which gets trapped in the spaces around the cells is the cause of fluid retention and increased pressure in the body, which results in pain, nutritive damage to the cells, premature old age, and even death. In short, trapped plasma protein is the major cause of degenerative disease in America today."

This lymphologist points out that as individuals and as a population we are keeping ourselves at low level wellness by eating too much of protein foods, causing the trapping of protein molecules within the interstitial fluid spaces.

Furthermore, trapped plasma protein "can be caused by negative emotions, shallow breathing, and lack of exercise! It can also be caused by too much salt, sugar, fat and certain other foods," he says.[6]

Trapped plasma protein in the spaces between the cells is blamed by West as the source of pain, loss of energy, and the onset of degenerative disease such as heart attack, stroke, cancer, glaucoma, hearing loss, cataracts, diabetes, kidney failure, and others. He says that such trapping will cause death within twenty-four hours because:

• Trapped plasma protein forces the cells away from the capillary membrane which results in lack of oxygen and nutrients to the cell.

• Trapped plasma protein causes fluid retention in the spaces around the cells.

• It leads to sickness and eventual death of the human organism.

---

[6]C. Samuel West. *Trapped Protein, The Major Cause of pain, loss of energy, and degenerative disease (a pamphlet). (Mesa, Arizona: The New Way of Life Health Foundation, January 1978), p. 2.*

• Trapped plasma protein attracts the positive sodium ion. Excess sodium in the spaces around the cells upsets the sodium-potassium balance (which should be in a ratio of one sodium to nine potassium ions), and this blocks the electrical activity of the cell. The cell is unable to take in nutrients from the blocking of electrical charges. Worse, it cannot give off its waste. Toxic material tends to build up and poisoning of the cells takes place. The cell will die. If enough cells die, the human organism dies.[7]

In 1961, Dr. Guyton discovered that the spaces around body cells have a negative sub-atmospheric pressure. This negative interstitial fluid pressure is explained by the fluid flowing into lymphatic vessels from interstitial spaces even when the mean interstitial fluid pressure is negative, because this pressure rises and falls every time a tissue is compressed, as discussed earlier. When the pressure rises to a value slightly above atmospheric pressure, fluid flows out of the interstitial spaces into the lymphatics. This illustrates how capillary dynamics and interstitial fluid pressure work together to keep you functioning at a near-normal state.

The scientist went on to tell how this intermittent movement of interstitial fluid into the lymphatics holds the protein concentration of the cellular liquid at a low value and thereby holds the interstitial colloid osmotic pressure at a low value, usually about 4 mm. Hg. With the tissue colloid osmotic pressure so low, the plasma colloid osmotic pressure becomes greatly preponderant, causing osmosis of so much additional fluid directly into the capillaries that the average pressure in the interstitial spaces is maintained at a very negative value of -7 mm. Hg.

Until the measurement was revised in 1971, Dr. Guyton originally measured this negative value at -6 mm Hg., and West has developed a "Health Education Program" which stresses the -6 mm Hg. concept.

---

[7]*Ibid.* p. 4.

The normal tendency for the capillaries to absorb fluid from the interstitial spaces tends to create a partial vacuum. This vacuum forces all the minute structures of the interstitial spaces to be compacted together. No excess fluid is present besides that required simply to fill the crevices between the tissue elements.

This so-called "dry" state of the tissue is particularly important for optimal nutrition of the tissues, since nutrients pass from the blood to the cells by diffusion; and the rate of diffusion between two points is inversely proportional to the distance between the cells and the capillaries. Therefore, it is essential that the distances be maintained at a minimum; otherwise, nutritive damage to the cells can result.[8]

The theory of the deleterious effects of excess protein leeched from the blood and into the tissue spaces may be summarized in a listing. West says in his lectures and writings that trapped plasma protein does the following:[9]

- It brings in too much sodium to the tissues.
- It blocks the circulation within the tissues spaces.
- It produces nutritional deficiencies in the cells.
- It causes unhealthy and swollen cells.
- It increases the pressure of the interstitial fluid.
- It produces pain (probably from lack of oxygen).
- It decreases the ability of the lymphatic system to neutralize and destroy the poisons produced by cellular waste.
- It short-circuits the electrical system of the body by allowing the accumulation of poisons.
- It drains the body of energy.
- It places a continual strain on the liver, kidneys, lungs, and skin to excrete the waste.
- It eventually blocks circulation to the muscle and pulls bones out of place by muscular spasm.

---

[8]Guyton (1971), *Op. cit.*, p. 190.

[9]C. Samuel West. *Excess Protein* (a brochure). (Mesa, Arizona: New Way of Life Health Institute, March 1977), p. iii.

• It decreases the efficient functioning of body organs in proportion to the amount of excess protein concentration they possess.

• It leads to sickness and eventual death of the human organism

In short, as the plasma proteins get trapped in the spaces around the cells, this lymphologist affirms, they alter the "dry" state of perfect health. In the dry state, there is no excess fluid present, only that which is necessary to fill the crevices around the cells. The plasma proteins in excess also alter the negative sub-atmospheric pressure, which holds the cells tightly and close to the capillary membrane, a condition which is necessary for the cells to receive sufficient oxygen and nutrients.[10]

Is Your Lymphatic System Working Well?

At the start of this chapter we said that the lymphatic system is the garbage can of your body. The less cluttered and more freely flowing the lymph channels are, the healthier you will tend to be. You'll heal more quickly in case of injury, clear up any organ imbalances with ease, and get rid of disease if the disposal of end products of metabolism are carried out without a hitch.

But how do you know how well your garbage disposal system is working? Is pain the primary symptom to govern yourself by? No! If you wait for pain to strike before taking stock of your lymphatic system, you've already waited too long.

The most apparent way to check the lymphatics is to merely look in the mirror at your eyes, skin, hair, nails, and posture. Noticing the latter first, the skeletal joints and how you hold yourself erect will tell you a lot. Bursitis being present in the shoulders or as bun-

---

[10]C. Samuel West. *Trapped Plasma Proteins* (a brochure). (Mesa, Arizona: The Dr. West Health Education Foundation, August 1978), p. i.

ions on the feet, stooped posture, rounded shoulders, and a crooked spine are declarations of a lymphatic circulation filled with toxicity and poor nutrition. Dry or arthritic joints are symptomatic of lymphatic imbalances. This is also true of the connective tissue throughout the entire body. The fascia isn't being nourished sufficiently if there is joint stiffness or soft tissue spasm. Then you'll know that very little of your waste products are being carried away efficiently from the cells.

Any of the apparent external characteristics such as drooping of eyelids, flaking of skin, breaking of nails, falling out of hair are indicators that poisons are present and not being expelled. Especially significant is bad breath and body odors of the feet and armpits. You may brush your teeth and wash a great deal and yet, still be offensive to others and cognizant of the odor to yourself. The reason there's a smell? Inadequate excretion of cellular waste, and large molecules of protein from the blood are likely to be trapped in the interstitial spaces.

The spinal fluid, which bathes the brain and spinal cord, is also essentially part of the lymphatic system. Its movement and replenishment are essential for a healthy central nervous system. When your lymphatics aren't functioning well, you're going to experience unclear thinking, lethargy, dull headaches, irritability, depression, anxiety, and the desire to sleep much of the time.

You might suffer from varicose veins, hemorrhoids, or a tendency for blood clots to form. These additionally come from blockage of the venous circulation. There is likely less lymph being allowed back into the full system at the critical subclavian vein junctures resulting from a sluggish venous return. This can produce toxicity and further stagnation of the blood flow.

What's needed is the very thing we are generally speaking of in this book, rebounding aerobics to stimulate an optimum drainage of the lymphatic circulation.

Such exercise, performed as it is against gravity, dilates the capillaries and allows greater blood flow throughout the tissues than when the body is at rest. No stagnation of fluids is allowed this way. Movement of blood stimulates the tissues by providing additional tissue fluid to speed through the interstitial spaces around the cells. Food and oxygen are carried in that fluid, which gives up its nourishment by osmosis. The lymph ducts dilate considerably during the aerobic bound, as well.

By rebounding, a true aerobic effect takes place — better aerobics than furnished by any other form of exercise. There is a general flushing of the cells with wastes given up to the cellular interstitial fluid. The waste-laden-liquid is carried away through the lymphatic tree of vessels until they empty into the subclavian veins and are unloaded from the body through action of the excretory organs, the lungs, skin, kidneys, and liver.

Last chapter item: The lymphatic and excretory organs do their job of getting rid of the body's garbage more efficiently when suitable quantities of water are present and are being excreted. About two or three quarts of water drunk each day does wonders for your lymphatic drainage system. Water, combined with instant aerobics from rebounding, provides a fine cellular and lymphatic cleansing.

5

Reduction of Mental Stress by Rebounding

Famous actress Julie Harris, skilled heart surgeon Norman B. Thompson, Jr., television producer Don Ohlmeyer, and airtraffic controller Sidney Finkelberg have something in common. All of them turn to physical exercise as a means of overcoming the mental or emotional stress that goes with their jobs.

Julie Harris has appeared in comedies, dramas and musicals for the stage, movies and TV, winning awards for *Member of the Wedding, I Am a Camera,* and *The Lark.* She says rehearsals for the theater are probably the most strenuous part of acting. During pre-Broadway, out-of-town trials, she works twelve hours or more at a stretch rehearsing all day to perfect lines, cues, timing, and costume changes. Then she performs at night. Dialogue is frequently changed after it's been painstakingly learned; even names of characters are changed. This is a repeated source of pressure.

Another pressure is the fear that she will fail. "My hands sweat, my whole body feels clammy, and I worry. Will the door open? Will the note be on the table? I even get to feeling I may go to pieces and have to be replaced!"

How does she counteract these various stresses? "Fresh air and exercise are helpful," she says, "even a walk around the block. When you do Shakespeare at Stratford, Ontario, there's a dart board backstage to provide diversion for the actors."[1]

Norman B. Thompson, Jr., M.D., Director of Cardio-thoracic Surgery at St. Francis Hospital in Roslyn, New York, has done pioneering work in cardiac surgery for children. He replaces coronary arteries and valves and corrects cardiac defects, sometimes in infants, and directs a sixteen-member operating-room team in operations that last up to thirteen hours. The tension is terrific.

"The tension doesn't just dissolve after surgery," says Dr. Thompson. "The next six hours, in Intensive Care, may be the most critical. There are so many unanswered questions. How much time did we have? How reliable was the heart-lung machine? How serious were chemical abnormalities in the patient?"

How does he face the pressure? Between operations he rids himself of tension and fatigue by going for a swim.[2]

Don Ohlmeyer, the producer of NFL Monday Night Football on ABC-TV, a telecast seen by forty million viewers each week, works twelve-hour days and is lucky to have dinner at home once a week.

While the game is being televised, between 9:00 P.M. and midnight, he sits at a console before twenty TV monitor screens in a control truck outside the stadium in whatever city the game is being played. He is plugged in by intercom headset to three announcers, a director and various engineers, technicians and assistants, to keep track of the work of ten cameramen. "There's more

---

[1] Neal Ashby. "People under pressure." *Physicians World* (Vol. II, No. 3., March 1974), p. 30.

[2] *Ibid.*, p. 31.

pressure in that truck once a week during the football season than 99.9 percent of the American people undergo in an entire week," Ohlmeyer estimates.

During the action, he fields over-the-shoulder suggestions from his executive producers, directs his staff, chooses which players to focus isolation shots on, worries about whether his people are doing anything to irritate NFL officials, and tells Howard Cosell when to profile a key player on the field.

How does he dissolve the tension and pressure? Ohlmeyer plays tennis with announcers Frank Gifford and Don Meredith the entire weekend before the Monday game, to relax before the stress hits him.[3]

As an air-traffic controller in the New York Air Route Traffic Control Center at Ronkonkoma, New York, Sidney Finkelberg spends his workday staring at a glowing, yellow radarscope, wearing a ground-to-air radio headset, and following and directing the movement of as many as thirty-two multi-million-dollar airplanes at a time in and out of the three busy New York City airports. He governs the life or death of thousands of passengers daily.

"We have plenty of pressure," says Finkelberg. "This is one of the busiest aircraft sectors in the country. And from time to time our work is complicated by bad weather. Thunderstorms are our nemesis. Aircraft may deviate 200 miles from their planned routes to avoid these storms."

How does such an air-traffic controller deal with stress? Finkelberg and his co-workers engage in vigorous sports. Rather than golf or bowl, they play basketball, softball, and tennis. "I doubt if any other profession has so many active athletes in their thirties and forties," he observes. "Exercise takes the mind completely off work and heats up and loosens the muscles that get cramped while you sit at the scope."[4]

---

[3]*Ibid.*, p. 31.

[4]*Ibid.*, p. 30.

What Stress Is and Does

All of us find ourselves daily in the midst of mentally stressful situations to one degree or another. An argument with a loved one, the deadliness and pressure of a career, the demands of hectic schedules — all of these can produce responses of anxiety, uncertainty, frustration, or anger. Along with them, we usually have characteristic physical reactions of rapid heartbeat, pounding headaches, soaring blood pressure, or other irregularities.

When mental stress becomes excessive — prolongs the body in constant tension and reaction — good health can be destroyed.

Your response to stress releases ACTH in the body from the adrenal cortex glands known as **corticotropins.** ACTH is adreno-coricotrophic hormone, a very imporant metabolizer that reduces the level of adrenal ascorbic acid and decreases adrenal cholesterol. This is what allows the body, whether it be man or animal, to adapt itself to any kind of stress.[5]

What could interfere with the production of ACTH, and thus cause disease from stress? Two things: lack of bodily movement in the form of routine exercise and nutritional deficiency of a particular type. While this is a book about rebounding exercise, let us provide you with a brief explanation of the nutrient factors connected with stress disease.

ACTH could be reduced in production by a lack of vitamins A or D or a deficiency in the minerals calcium, magnesium, or phosphorus. These various nutrients usually consumed in the diet must be present because they help stimulate the pituitary gland at the base of the brain. The pituitary gland, in turn, tells the adrenal gland to issue the "fight or flight" hormone adrenaline. A deficiency of these vitamins or minerals means that the

---

[5]Joseph Fruton and Sofia Simmonds. *General Biochemistry.* New York: John Wiley & Sons, Inc., 1953, p. 467.

pituitary cannot supply the body with enough ACTH to activate the adrenals. The stress situation cannot be confronted and adapted; therefore, illness will result.

One way to prevent the stimulation of stress disease is to supplement the diet with suitable quantities of nutrients. It is a means of preventing and even reversing degenerative disease such as cancer, stroke, hardening of the arteries, diabetes, glaucoma, and others.[6]

As an aside, let us point out that people of the Western industrialized countries often subject themselves to gastrointestinal stress by the eating of badly cooked foods, insufficient raw foods, irritation from chemical processing of food, overly refined foods, sugar, artificial forms of edibles, irregular meals including starvation diets for weight loss, fad diets, drugs, alcohol, and other things swallowed. We'll have more to say about why, how, and what the American people eat as they do in this book's last chapter.

A prime example of gastrointestinal stress is the ingestion by Americans of countless drug preparations and various newly discovered remedies. We stress ourselves with drugs. If we are lucky, our bodies may withstand the onslaught of chemicals and miraculously return to health. Of course, there is always a risk involved that the drug will produce more distress and discomfort than the original disorder it was intended to cure.

The American College of Physicians and the U.S. Food and Drug Administration readily admit that even the best drug is capable of causing harmful side effects in susceptible persons. Such drugs are definitely stressors. "Three to five percent of the hospitalization in the United States is a result of adverse drug reaction, and approximately 30,000 died from it last year," said Dr. Wayne Evans, director of the Massachusetts College

---

[6]Andre Voisin. *Soil, Grass and Cancer.* London: Cosby, Lockwood & Son, Ltd., 1959, p. 226.

of Pharmacy's Center for Citizen Health Learning.[7]

At the University of Montreal, Hans Selye, M.D., Ph.D., D.Sc., in the 1920's and 1930's added greatly to our current understanding of stress and how it affects the adrenal glands. He defined stress as the ordinary and extraordinary pressures of life that confront every individual. These pressures cause varying reactions that may be psychological or physiological or both and are involved in the way we cope with the pressures of life. Stress begins with the pressure, the daily routines, responsibilities and chores that keep us going, usually in some kind of work schedule or what might be called a "social harness" — stable expectations guiding or harnessing both work and recreation. These activities are the normal pressures of life — far too loosely called the normal stresses of life.

However, there is a fundamental difference between pressure and stress. Pressure is a stimulus — external or internal — to which we respond. Stress results from our perception of the need and our gearing up for the response. It's a coupled response. Thus, the need to arise from a sleep at a particular time is the pressure. The stress, if there from arising too late and having to rush, is derived from the way we perceive and respond to this pressure of wakefulness. A more functional term to describe this kind of pressure is "stressor." And stress, if it occurs, is in response to the stressor.

Dr. Selye has described the general adaptation syndrome (GAS) that is characteristic of stress. It consists of three stages: the alarm reaction, the resistance stage, and exhaustion. The alarm reaction is a call on the body's defensive mechanism — provided by the adrenal gland, already described. The alarm reaction is present during any stress, which can be of an emotional nature, a physical injury, a chemical stress in the form of food additives, thermal stress with exposure to temperature

---

[7]"How common medicines work: a crash course for laymen." *The Advocate,* July 25, 1977, p. 11.

change, mental duress, a demand to fight, or other situations.

The second portion of the general adaptation syndrome is the resistance stage when the stress which activated the alarm reaction is present for a prolonged period. The adrenal gland actually grows in size to meet the demand of this long-term stress.

The third part of the GAS is the exhaustion stage, which is when the adrenal becomes depleted and functional hypoadrenia sets in. Then, because you have no more adrenaline with which to react to the stressor — you can't cope and become ill. Lingering in the exhaustion stage can kill.

Functional hypoadrenia has so many symptoms that many doctors not knowledgeable in its diagnosis and treatment have classified patients with this condition as psychosomatic, hypochondriac, or as having a "nervous" condition, and give them tranquilizers.

A Significant Survey on Exercising Out of Stress

In June, 1979 the American Academy of Family Physicians conducted a survey of the lifestyles and personal health care in different occupations. The study was designed to examine and compare the attitudes and practices of six occupational groups representing differing social, educational and economic circumstances — business executives, family physicians, farmers, garment workers, secretaries, and teachers.

A wide spectrum of health and lifestyle questions were distributed by Research & Forecasts, Inc., of New York City which were answered by 4,500 people in these six occupations. Questions on exercise were among them. In large measure, exercise was a tool to help the six groups cope with stress in their lives. In fact, family physicians and business executives noted their reliance on exercise as a means of coping with stress, at least 50 percent of the time. Farmers declared themselves as getting plenty of exercise and didn't list this method separately. But 30 percent of teachers, 26 percent of the secretaries, and 25 percent of the garment workers use specific programs of exercise as the way to cope.

Two questions asked of these people were: "Do you believe exercise is important to your health?" "How often do you engage in physical exercise outside of work?"

Belief in the importance of exercise to good health was nearly unanimous, ranging from 86 percent of the garment workers to 95 percent of the physicians. Only 3 percent of the garment workers said that exercise is *not* important; the remaining 11 percent said they are not sure. Only 1 percent of the physicians, executives, teachers or secretaries were ready to say "no" to the question on exercise, making this the health issue on which there is far and away the least disagreement.

Nonetheless, less than half of the farmers, garment workers, and secretaries and only slightly more than half of the teachers claimed to exercise twice a week or more. About two-thirds of the doctors and executives declared they do so.

When asked to indicate which types of exercise they actually engage in, all six groups were in agreement on the number one activity: walking. Walking is two to three times as popular as any other form of exercise.

The second most popular form of exercise varied from group to group. For physicians, it is jogging; for executives and teachers, calisthenics. For farmers it is their work itself. For garment workers as for secretaries, the second most popular form of exercise is dancing.

If a 20 percent response rate is taken as an arbitrary cutoff point (i.e., 20 percent or more of the respondents indicating their involvement in a given form of exercise), executives appear to get the greatest variety of physical activity. They checked off six forms of exercise: walking, calisthenics, jogging, golf, tennis, and swimming. Farmers and garment workers get the least variety; 20 percent of them checking only two activities: walking and dancing for garment workers and walking and working for farmers. Physicians and teachers followed close upon the executives at five choices each. Physicians prefer walking, jogging, bicycling, swimming, and golf. Teachers engage in walking, calisthenics, bicycling, swimming, and dancing. Secretaries indicated substantial involvement in four forms of exercise: walking, dancing, calisthenics, and bicycling.

Because of significant differences between men and women on the question of "what types of exercise do you do?" the choices are for "men only" among the executives, physicians, and farmers; for "women only" among garment workers, secretaries, and teachers.

Tennis showed up on this survey list only once, that of the executives. Golf and jogging are indulged in by 20 percent or more of only the physicians and executives. A certain amount of faddishness may account for some of these patterns; economic considerations may account for others. The presence of dancing on the lists of all three groups which are primarily female may also suggest a gender-based preference. Note that physicians, teachers, and secretaries enjoy cycling; executives, teachers, and secretaries enjoy calisthenics. Swimming appeals to physicians, executives, and teachers; dancing enchants teachers, garment workers, and secretaries. "Team sports" are not popular with any of the six groups under study — an 8 percent response rate from teachers being the highest.

It may be obvious to anyone regularly using the rebounder that these six occupational groups are missing out on an excellent method of exercise. We believe the reason they don't engage in routine rebounding aerobics is that they haven't yet been apprised of the existence of rebounding devices and the new science of *reboundology. Undoubtedly the anti-stress benefits of rebounding will reach them eventually.

---

*See p. iii.

Specific Anti-stress Benefits of Rebounding

Reduction of mental stress by rebounding has been proven over and over again by scientific studies. Stress research in the United States centers on heart disease, and for good reason. Cardiovascular ailments such as coronary heart disease now take an appalling annual toll in lives of American men in vigorous middle age. Of the 1,000,000 people who died from coronary heart disease in the U.S. last year, almost one-third were under sixty-five.

In fact, for those who are recovering from a heart attack, the recommendation often is to exercise. Doctors believe that for most patients exercise is beneficial, provided it does not cause pain, shortness of breath, or other symptoms. The patient should not engage in exercise until he discusses his limitations with his physician, including the desirability of special testing for the amount of stress he can tolerate.

Research is going on constantly, and all forms of investigations are being used. The latest is exercising pigs. The pigs are jogging in an Arizona State University study on the effects of exercise and high-fat diets on heart problems. A graduate student in agriculture, Ross Consaul, and George Seperich, an assistant professor of agriculture, head the study that has their pigs running two miles a day.

Mr. Consaul jogs behind the pigs, occasionally prodding them with a long two-pronged fork, to keep up the pace. "They burn up the track for about the first lap," he said. "After that, most of them need some encouragement. We started them with a nice, easy jog most people could do — about a third of a mile. Then, as soon as they improve their time by 10 percent, we increase their distance by 50 meters."

The pigs were chosen for the study because many of their psychological characteristics resemble those of humans, such as susceptibility to stress and heart attacks.

Pigs were also chosen because, as Professor Seperich put it, "We can be fairly sure no one is going to invite our pigs out for beer and pizza in the middle of our study."

There are eighteen pigs involved. Six have jogged daily since they were forty-pound piglets; six started jogging after they reached the middle-age weight of 150 pounds, and six simply sit around eating and sleeping in the usual pig fashion. They are separated into normal and well-balanced diet groups, high in saturated fats, and high in unsaturated fats.

The two researchers have found the jogging pigs are more energetic and cheerful than the sedentary ones. They seem to suffer less from stress.[8]

Prior research with exercise has turned up more than thirty particular benefits from regular movement in either one's occupation, recreation, or for purposes of just bodily motion. The specific anti-stress benefits of rebounding are even more exaggerated, since, as Albert E. Carter points out in his book, *The Miracles of Rebound Exercise,* "Rebounding not only increases the strength of each muscle by increasing the G force repeatedly, but also increases the fitness of the muscle by improving lymphatic and blood circulation in the muscle."[9]

The following are thirty specific anti-stress benefits of performing rebounding aerobics on a regular basis:[10]

1) It tones up the glandular system to increase the output of the thyroid gland, the pituitary gland, and the adrenals. The thyroid's hormonal production stimulates or affects almost every important body process, including the body's use of oxygen. The pituitary stimulates, regulates, and coordinates the functions of the other

---

[8]"Jogging pigs get in step." *The New York Times,* May 27, 1980, p. 43.

[9]Albert E. Carter. *The Miracles of Rebound Exercise.* (Bothell, Washington: The National Institute of Reboundology & Health, 1979), p. 88.

[10]Morton Walker. *How Not to Have a Heart Attack.* (New York: Franklin Watts, Inc., 1980), pp. 203 & 204.

endocrines. For this reason, the pituitary gland is called the master gland of the body. The two main functions of the hormones of the adrenal cortex are the control of the proper salt and water content of the body; and the regulation of carbohydrate, fat, and protein metabolism. In addition, the adrenal cortex secretes sex hormones, mainly androgens, similar to those produced by the testicles.

2) It strengthens the heart and any other muscle being used in the body so that the muscle works more efficiently. Muscle tissue is made up of elastic cells and fibers that can repeatedly contract and relax. Whenever we move, we do so by contraction of some particular set of muscles attached to the skeleton. When we hold ourselves erect against gravity we are using muscles in opposing groups, some held in a contracted state in order to maintain our balance. Increase the G force, and you will cause greater contraction — the involved muscles work harder and get stronger. Rebounding increases the G force at the bottom of each bounce.

3) By strengthening the heart muscle, it allows the resting heart to beat less often. Each beat becomes more powerful and sends out a greater surge of blood around the body to nourish its 60 trillion cells.

4) It encourages collateral circulation, the formation of new branch blood vessels that distribute blood to the heart muscle and to other body parts by alternate routes. This indirect, subsidiary or accessory influx of new blood supply is valuable when there is a lack of nutrition to the tissues as the result of impairment of the main blood flow.

5) It tends to reduce the height to which the arterial pressure rises during exertion. The same kind of training effect that occurs from aerobics performance with external muscles, takes place in the media, or middle muscle layer of the arteries. The training effect gives the media greater muscle tone, and elevation of the blood pressure becomes less great in time of stress.

6) Furthermore, the blood pressure won't remain

elevated quite so long because of this training effect, and it lessens the time during which the blood pressure remains below normal after severe activity. The blood pressure drops suddenly after the need for its elevation is removed; the training effect from rebounding aerobics brings up the dropped pressure to its normal level more quickly.

7) It lowers elevated cholesterol and triglyceride levels. As indicated in chapter two, L. Howard Harley, M.D., Director of Exercise at Beth Israel Hospital and Associate Professor of Medicine, Harvard Medical School, discussed the relationship between physical activity and other risk factors for heart disease at a symposium sponsored by The American Heart Association, October 18, 1978. Dr. Hartley said, "Exercise can have a direct effect on blood lipids," and studies have shown that "people who exercise regularly reduce their levels of serum cholesterol and serum triglycerides." Results of studies have also shown that exercise increases levels of high density lipoprotein fraction of cholesterol and "all of these effects of exercise are expected to have a favorable effect on cardiovascular health maintenance," said the exercise physiologist.

8) It holds off the incidence of cardiovascular disease. This is evident by acknowledging the risk factors of high blood pressure, high cholesterol, high triglycerides, high LDL (low density lipoprotein) and realizing that rebounding exercises reduce all of these elevated readings that have your heart at risk.

9) It increases the functional activity of the red bone marrow in the production of red blood cells. The red blood cells carry oxygen and nutrients to the tissues of the body and also help remove carbon dioxide from them. They are formed in the cancellous portion of the bone, the red marrow of which consists largely of blood corpuscles in all stages of development. About five million mature red blood cells are produced and released into the bloodstream every second. The blood platelets, which are essential for blood clot formation, and the white

blood cells, which protect the body against infection, are also formed in the red marrow.

10) It establishes a better equilibrium between the oxygen required by the tissues and the oxygen made available. This equilibrium is established by the red cells in the blood that carry oxygen to the organs and tissues and remove the carbon dioxide from them.

11) It circulates more oxygen to the tissues. The different oxygen and carbon dioxide concentrations in the blood in the capillaries, and in the air in the alveoli cause the two to exchange gases. Carbon dioxide, at a higher concentration in the blood, leaves it and enters the lungs. Oxygen, which initially has a higher concentration in the lungs, leaves them and enters the blood. In the blood, oxygen combines with the red coloring matter, hemoglobin, which transports it, pumped by the heart, to all the organs and tissues in the body.

12) It increases the capacity for respiration. Breathing is controlled by changes in the volume of the chest cavity, brought about mainly by muscular movements of the diaphragm. Expansion and contraction of the lungs to fill the cavity result in lower and higher air pressures within them, which are equilized with the atmospheric pressure as air is forced into and out of the lungs. Repeated rebounding aerobics accomplishes more muscular movements of the diaphragm with the consequent chest expansion.

13) It causes muscles to perform work in moving fluids through the body — which lightens the load on the heart. With two-thirds of the body comprised of liquids, the ability to send fluid to areas where it is needed such as to sites of inflammation, becomes vital. The amount of fluid in the body remains constant, controlled by the workings of the kidneys, and the surplus is disposed of through the bladder, lungs, intestines, and skin. The muscles also help in this disposal effort.

14) It aids lymphatic circulation, as well as the flow in the veins of the circulatory system. Lymph is pushed through the lymphatic system by contractions of the ves-

sel walls, by differences in pressure, and by the movements of muscles in surrounding parts of the body. At
the base of the neck, the two main branches of the lymphatic system merge with two veins, and the lymph becomes part of the bloodstream.

15) It promotes body growth and repair. Growth of
the long bones are especially stimulated by rebounding;
this is true because of the stimulative effect on the pituitary gland. The gland's frontal lobe produces at least
six necessary hormones, one of which is the growth-
stimulating hormone.

16) It stimulates metabolism, which is a complex and
continuous process that begins in the digestive tract and
the lungs and goes on in every cell of the body. It consists of breaking down substances into simpler parts that
are then recombined into countless new substances that
compose the body. Every one of these chemical changes
either uses up or releases energy, and rebounding conditions all the body's systems to handle energy more
efficiently.

17) It enhances digestion and elimination processes.
The beginning of metabolism is digestion, where food
is broken down into simpler elements so that it may be
absorbed into the bloodstream and used for energy,
repair of tissues, and growth. The end products of digestion are eliminated from the body and regular musculalr
activity carries the entire process forward effectively.

18) It expands the capacity for fuel storage, causing
extra endurance. But the storage will be as deposits of
protein rather than fat because of the extra muscular
motion from rebounding.

19) It reduces the likelihood of obesity, for exercise
is vital in taking off excess weight. A daily program of
rebounding aerobics may not cause the pounds to melt
away overnight, but it will diminish body fat, improve
muscle tone, improve the efficiency with which your body
burns carbohydrates, and lower your pulse rate and
blood pressure. Remember, there are 150 calories in
a glass of beer. If your body does not need the energy

these calories provide, and if you don't want the beer to end up as fatty tissue, you will have to rebound for two minutes,[11] run for six minutes, swim for 10 minutes, or walk for 22 minutes in order to burn up the extra calories.

20) It provides an addition to the alkaline reserve of the body which may be of significance in an emergency requiring prolonged effort. The principal acid neutralizer, or base, in the body is sodium bicarbonate, which is manufactured from carbon dioxide and from sodium obtained from dietary salt. Sodium bicarbonate helps to maintain the delicate balance between acidity and alkalinity that is necessary for the normal chemical activity in the body. By stimulating metabolism, rebounding enhances this whole alkaline mechanism.

21) It more nearly attains absolute potential of the cells through chemical function. Cells respond to stimuli from the environment outside their walls. They perform the special task designed for them in the total economy of the living body. Thus, they will live up to their potential and function at peak performance if the environment is ideal. Oxygenation by muscular movement to increase respiration and circulation permit this potential.

22) It improves coordination through the transmission of more impulses and responsiveness of the muscle fibers. Impulses travel along a nerve by a series of reactions that are partly chemical, partly electrical. Motor, or efferent, neurons carry impulses from the central nervous sytem to the various parts of the body, where they are translated into action. At the outer end of a motor neuron, the frayed end of an axon spreads out to form an end plate, which connects with muscle fibers. Similar structures at the ends of sensory nerves are concentrated in the sense organs and irregularly dispersed in the skin. The more coordinated procedures

---

[11]Figures presented in the lecture, "Techniques of Exercise Testing The Obese Patient" by Paul E. DeVore, M.D. given at American Society of Bariatric Physicians, March 1979.

are carried out, the finer becomes future coordination efforts. Rebounding is a coordinative process.

23) It affords a feeling of muscular vigor from increased muscle tone. Healthy muscles are important to our sense of well-being, our grace, coordination, and energy. But only properly exercised muscles stay in good condition; the reduced muscle tone that goes with a sedentary life can lead to poor circulation and a sense of physical depression. If muscles are not used at all because of prolonged bedrest or other immobilization, they become weak and atrophied.

24) It supplies a reserve of bodily strength and physical efficiency. Even when we stand perfectly still, muscles are at work supporting our weight and maintaining our balance. While we sleep the muscles of our internal organs continue their motions. Stored within the belly of a muscle is protein and sometimes fat that comes forth when called upon to provide hidden quantities of strength and energy.

25) It offers relief from neck and back pains, from headaches, and from other pains caused by lack of use of the various joints and muscles of the body. Almost everyone has experienced a charley horse that results from too violent use of a muscle. The muscle protests against an unaccustomed activity by becoming sore, stiff, and painful. By rebounding regularly, it's not likely you'll ever again have a charley horse.

26) It curtails the occurrence of fatigue and menstrual discomforts for women. Muscles are affected by a great variety of disorders. They also are the underlying cause of many health problems. Fatigue, overwork of a group of muscles, nervousness, or insomnia, for example, bring on muscle twitches and spasms. The same is true of muscle cramps, especially those in the lower abdomen which may be related to dysmenorrhea or other female trouble.

27) It results in better mental performance, with keener learning processes. You can help your brain to stay healthy and work at top efficiency by providing

it with the necessary diversion through exercise and the sufficient amount of sleep it requires. Much movement will bring on good sleep.

28) It allows for better and easier relaxation and sleep. The amount of sleep needed differs with individuals, but generally the body and mind tell you they are tired. If anxiety or discomfort are interfering with your sleep, a good session of rebounding aerobics does wonders to give you the necessary relaxation diversion.

29) It minimizes the numbers of colds, allergies, digestive disturbances, and abdominal problems. Simply, rebounding keeps the entire body with all its variable systems in tune. They work coordinately to provide optimum metabolism.

30) It tends to stop premature aging. The effects of hardening of the arteries are reversed, prevented, or diminished. By conquering this ultimate pathology of the main degenerative diseases you will keep your mind alert, skin smooth, skeleton flexible, libido intact, kidneys functioning, blood circulating, liver detoxifying, enzyme systems alive, hold onto your memory, and avoid different symptoms of the aging process. Rebounding aerobics will do it all for you. It offers limberness, pliability, strength, and stretch for all parts of the body. It does away with "desk-bound flabbiness" and executive stress which sometimes is the fate of many business executives and other persons.

Peter Houck, President of Houck Industries, Inc. of Tulare, California, was one such business executive who was introduced to rebounding aerobics. As a manufacturer of metal drawer runners with nylon bearings, Mr. Houck first observed exercises on a rebounding device at a home furnishings show. He read *The Miracles of Rebound Exercise* and later was again put in touch with rebounding by seeing a demonstration of it at his civic organization. He bought a rebound unit for himself and worked with the unit faithfully.

Seeing the benefits of rebounding on his own body, Houck decided this was something his factory employees would enjoy, as well. Consequently, he wrote to Albert Carter and asked what it would take to persuade Carter to travel to Tulare to explain in person exactly what rebounding exercise was.

Houck purchased six rebound units and six weeks later Carter presented rebounding aerobics to the entire staff of Houck Industries. In a lecture to each of two groups, forty employees in one and twenty in another, Carter gave a full description and demonstration.

Two weeks later, Peter Houck bought forty more rebound units. Two weeks after that, he ordered another six units, a total of fifty-two besides the one he used at home. Why? Because this business executive noticed a marked reduction in stress reactions among his employees from their engaging in rebound exercise. Production increased; people showed improved physical capabilities; they had uplifted spirits; felt more at peace; required fewer hours for sleeping; generally looked healthier; acted more cheerfully at the workplace; a reduction in absenteeism took place; and pulse rates and blood pressures of employees who were tested all reduced in readings.

Peter Houck noticed that he personally took firmer control of stress situations arising from his business enterprise. Whenever he felt nervous tension, he'd slip off his shoes to rebound for ten minutes or so. His administrative decisions became more effective, and he frequently arrived at them in the midst of his rebounding. Houck's investment in rebounding aerobics for himself and his employees brought a profitable return to the business.

6

Effects of Exercise on the Aging Process

"We suggest that you should use it or lose it," says C. Carson Conrad, executive director of the President's Council on Physical Fitness and Sports. "If you just sit around, you can watch bones and muscles atrophy. If you sit around and wait to die, you won't have to wait long."

The President's Council is making a concerted effort to get elderly people out of their chairs and into some healthful exercise programs. It's a chore of re-education for those over sixty-five, because, Conrad points out, "So many older people were busy making a living when they were young that they never had time for exercise. They looked on exercise as play, something for the children. Few had physical fitness programs when they were in school and even fewer took part in organized sports."[1]

As a result, statistics on the elderly and their exercising make dreary reading. When a National Adult

---

[1] Edward Edelson. "Exercise for elders." *Sunday News Magazine,* March 25, 1979, pp. 10 & 11.

Physical Fitness Survey was taken in March 1979, it found that nearly half of all adult Americans do not exercise, and the numbers were particularly poor for those aged fifty and over.

Yet, as we get older, we must do everything possible to resist the urge to slow down our lives' tempo. Complacency can kill! And a lack of desire to exercise is a form of complacency. Your well-exercised body will hold onto its flexibility and tone for all of your years if you'll use it and not let it corrode from non-movement.

Unfortunately, you're reading this at a time when many of us in middle age and older are already suffering with body disuse. The ridiculous rationale of non-exercisers is usually that extra body movement might bring on heart attacks or strained muscles, as we mentioned in chapter two. This reasoning is sheer nonsense and merely an excuse for their laziness. The fact is, only one percent or less of all heart attacks ever occur during exercise — usually among weekend athletes who exert themselves unwisely during hot summer days, or among winter snow-shovellers who have taken a hiatus from regular exercise.

So, to keep fit and stay young, do some sensible exercise, with the consent of your physician. Maybe it won't be an Olympic training program that puts undue stress on your body, but perform some brisk physical activity like rebounding aerobics every day.

Former screen Tarzan and Olympic swimming champion Johnny Weissmuller does just that. At age eighty-three, and headquartered at the International Hall of Fame, Inc. in Fort Lauderdale, Florida, he used his rebounding device daily. When he was age sixty-nine, Weissmuller had broken his hip and was informed he would be confined to using crutches for almost a year. After exercising on his rebound unit routinely for a month, he was able to dispose of the crutches and felt terrific. It had even reduced varicose veins in both of his legs.

"I feel it has restored fantastic circulation and lung capacity and muscle tone in my body. It is like having a complete gymnasium in my home," said Johnny Weissmuller. "In my opinion, this new rebound unit is the most effective training device any athlete could use. In fact, I believe every home should have at least one to stimulate physical fitness for the entire family."

Johnny Weissmuller knew what he was talking about because rebounding had helped to keep his body young. It prevents the crosslinkage reactions that bring on aging. Rebounding holds back the aging process.

The Crosslinkage Theory of Aging

Before, 1940, thousands of papers had been written about crosslinking as a means of stabilizing macromolecules for industrial purposes — for example, tanning hides to make them insoluble and resistant to microbial attack, and vulcanizing rubber to increase its stability. Controlled artificial crosslinking of gelatin made the photographic film possible. But no one had yet connected this vast body of knowledge with the changes that occur with the passage of time in collagen, elastin, and other large, reactive, biological molecules in the human body. Still, crosslinkage is well-accepted now as the true molecular and cellular basis for people growing old too soon.

What is crosslinkage? Crosslinkage reactions in the human body can attack and damage deoxyribonucleic acid and ribonucleic acid, the key substances that carry the genetic code. Deoxyribonucleic acid (DNA) and ribonucleic acid (RNA) determine what kinds of proteins a cell makes, and the kinds of proteins it makes determine how the cell behaves.

Chemical damage to DNA produces alterations called mutations in which cells may not be able to grow and divide normally; they may produce defective proteins, or become cancerous and give rise to tumors. Much of the cell damage that goes along with aging is due to accumulated mutations.

Crosslinkage reactions result in the union of at least two large molecules. A bridge or link between these is usually formed by a crosslinking agent; a small, motile molecule or free radical with a reactive hook or some other mechanism at both ends, capable of reacting with at least two large molecules. It is also possible for two large molecules to become crosslinked by the action of their own side chains or reactive groups present on one or both of them, or pathologically formed by ionizing radiation.[2]

In 1937, having studied under Nobel laureates Hans von Euler and A.I. Virtanen, Johan Bjorksten, Ph.D., now of the Bjorksten Research Foundation of Madison, Wisconsin, began directing a group working on stabilizing industrial protein gels in graphic arts. In 1942, he became famous in gerontology by expressing the crosslinkage theory of aging as follows:

> The aging of living organisms I believe is due to the occasional formation, by tanning, of bridges between protein molecules, which cannot be broken by the cell enzymes. Such irreparable tanning may be caused by tanning agents foreign to the organism or formed by unusual biological side reactions, or it may be due to the formation of a tanning bridge in some particular position in the protein molecule. In either event, the result is that cumulative tanning of body proteins, which we know as old age.[3]

If today we added the words "and nucleic acids" to "proteins," this concept of Bjorksten's still covers the basic tenets of the crosslinkage theory of aging. Indeed, it applies to any large molecule that contains sites reactive with sites on any crosslinking agent to which it can be exposed under physiologic conditions. One of the main physiologic conditions for crosslinking to take place is lack of exercise.

---

[2]Johan Bjorksten. "Crosslinkage and the aging process," in Rockstein, M (ed): *Theoretical Aspects of Aging*. (New York: Academic Press, 1974), pp. 43-53.

[3]Johan Bjorksten. "Chemistry of duplication." *Chem Ind* 50:69, 1942.

The theory is that crosslinkage is responsible for most of the secondary and tertiary causes of aging. While many previous conceptions about aging have been discredited, the crosslinkage theory has withstood the test of time.

We met with Dr. Bjorksten and discussed his crosslinkage theory at the semi-annual meeting of the American Academy of Medical Preventics, in Chicago, in May 1979. He stressed the significance of cross-linkages as a primary cause of many aging processes including atherosclerosis, failure of the immune system, loss of elasticity, decline in the secretion of many hormones, and increase in the sensitivity to trauma. Thus, if crosslinkage can be prevented or countered, a great many other conditions will be beneficially affected, including the prognosis of any disease in the older age brackets.

When asked how a person could prevent crosslinkage and slow down the aging process, Dr. Bjorksten admitted that the occurrence of unwanted random crosslinking cannot be avoided. "The crosslinking agents normally present in the human body are far too numerous and reactive," he said. "The reactions are too diverse to make practical any form of blockage and prevention of crosslinking reactions. However, some mitigation is possible."

He named five items of vital importance to mitigate the aging process. Without them, you will age very quickly and never approach the full complement of mankind's 120 possible years of life. These five components are abundantly present in the environment of long-lived people such as the residents of the village of Vilcabamba in what is called the Sacred Valley of a remote and rugged mountainous area of Ecuador. These residents, known as **Los Viejos** (Spanish for oldsters), thrive on the five necessary components for a long and healthy life: (1) an easy and relaxed attitude toward life with no emotional stress; (2) a natural, unprocessed diet of more raw foods and few cooked foods; (3) pure, fresh air with a fractionally higher oxygen content; (4) clean, clear, crystalline spring water loaded with mineral nutrients; and (5) vigorous, continuous, daily bodily movements for the accomplishment of work and play. Inasmuch as this book is focused on movement by rebounding, we shall detail the effects of exercise training on aging. Realize, however, that continuous movement of the muscles in aerobic actions is just one of five necessary components in the peaceful valley of the Ecuadorian Andes, where the residents enjoy health and freedom from premature aging matched only by the Hunzas of Pakistan and the Abkhazians of southern Russia.

Los Viejos and Their Way of Long Life

Vilcabamba is an ecologist's dream. It lies 4,500 feet above sea level and its water is provided by two sparkling rivers, the Uchima and the Chamba. The soil is rich in vitamins and minerals so that, for the most part, farming is carried on without chemicals. The clear mountain air is pure and sunlight streams into the town unhampered by industrial pollution.

We received this description of the Sacred Valley of the Andes from our colleague and fellow member of the American Society of Journalists and Authors, Inc., Grace Halsell. She visited there and lived with the residents, whom she remarked on as being peaceful, courteous, cheerful, and helpful to each other. Seldom does anyone raise his voice or become anxious over any situation. Grace learned that the village of Vilcabamba had an almost unbelievable number of people above the age of 100 years. While the United States has only three centenarians per 100,000 population, the Sacred Valley boasts nine in a population of less than 1,000. Also, Vilcabamba has no automobiles, no television and few radios. With no doctors, no hospitals and no health care system, the town is still known as an "island of immunity". The people don't get sick, and they live beyond 120 years in many instances.

Twenty percent of the reason for this, as we stated,

is that the residents exercise vigorously. Grace told us the people work hard. "Through stern physical labor all of their lives — not just to age sixty-two or sixty-five — they have earned for themselves a self-respect and sense of fulfillment missing in many urban lives. They are as one with the soil, or native to the earth as a seed of corn. Nature's cycle governs their lives from the green promise of spring to the mature ripeness of autumn. Age has mellowed and enriched them."

Grace told the whole of Los Viejos' story in an inspiring book.[4]

Since they are poor people and have no horses or burros, cars, or bikes to move them from one place to another, they walk everywhere, no matter how far, and put in long days farming. Their lives on foot exemplify the old saying that each of us has two doctors — the left and right legs. Los Viejos give their two doctors long and vigorous daily workouts, and they do this climbing steep mountain paths.

Rugged and vigorous, the people remain active into their 100's. It's thousands of miles from Vilcabamba to your home and ours. Can we in our society benefit from the examples of Los Viejos and still remain where we live? Most assuredly.

Before he died at the age of ninety-six in December 1977, Paul C. Bragg, Ph.D., N.D., R.Ph.T., the life extension specialist, author and lecturer whose permanent residence was in Hawaii on Waikiki Beach, used to emulate the actions of Los Viejos. Dr. Bragg performed rebounding aerobics every day from the time he was introduced to the rebound exercise unit when he was ninety-three years old. He rebounded for approximately thirty minutes daily and declared, "It has improved my stamina, endurance, and coordination besides improving my physical fitness, and strength. I wholeheartedly recommend the rebound unit to people

---

[4]Grace Halsell. *Los Viejos*. (Emmaus, Pennsylvania: Rodale Press, 1976).

of all ages as the finest exercising equipment in the entire world."

Paul Bragg engaged in rebounding aerobics specifically for the training effect such exercising had on slowing down the aging process.

Physiological Effect of Training on Aging

The major benefit of exercise is its effect on retarding the process of atherosclerosis. Muscular metabolism, especially the kind from vigorous use of the leg muscles during rebounding, acts to prevent hardening and clogging of the arteries. Also, as we have stated, rebounding causes bone marrow to increase production of red blood cells, while sedentary bone marrow becomes lazy and inactive.

Dr. Bjorksten told us that stroke, arteriosclerosis, circulatory disease, thrombosis, and heart disease are all different facets of the same crosslinking process. "Some injury causing increased permeability of the intima [the innermost layer of the arteries] is often an early occurrence . . . The circulating blood plasma normally contains crosslinking agents which over the years induce loss of elasticity. This loss of elasticity, or embrittlement, which is inherent in multiple crosslinkage, is most strongly evident in the elastic tissues.

"In the early years of life the loss of elasticity is not so evident, but sooner or later this loss will have progressed so far that the media [middle arterial layer] yields less readily than before to the recurrent pressures of the pulse wave," said Dr. Bjorksten. "The reduced yielding results in a larger force being required to effect the necessary displacement. Blood pressure rises, but even before this becomes evident, the intima is exposed to a hydrostatic stress at each heart beat. This stress increases progressively as the media hardens. The intima is thus exposed every second to a hydrostatic squeeze between the hardening media and the noncompressible circulating blood." The result? Hardening of the arteries.

How do you prevent this arterial hardening? Keep the bloodstream moving to avoid particulate matter such as blood corpuscles, chylomicrons, and other substances from being deposited in the subintimal region. You don't want these deposits. Otherwise, ingrowth of cells into the artery's central tunnel, the lumen, will occur. This is the start of the well-known atherosclerotic plaque that blocks almost all the arteries eventually.

To keep the bloodstream moving you have to engage the services of your two alternative "heart pumps" located in your calf muscles. The moving, contracting gastrocnemius, soleus, and plantaris calf muscles are proven to pump the blood up the circulatory tree through the veins and back to the heart and lungs for oxygenation and recirculation.

Roy J. Shephard, M.D., Ph. D., professor in the Department of Preventive Medicine and Biostatistics at the University of Toronto, and Terence Kavanagh, M.D., medical director of the Toronto Rehabilitation Medicine Center, University of Toronto, showed the value of such calf moving and whole body training among elderly participants in the age-specific Masters Athletic Competitions. They studied competitors in the 1975 World Masters Championships. Such competitors typically began their physical activity in the middle years and exercise with increasing vigor to an advanced age. These people thus offer insight into the effects of continued training on the aging process.

The two physicians learned that exercise can make participants feel more alive and less tense. Fatigue, one of the most universal signs of aging, is usually just the body's response to disuse. The Masters Athletic competitors did not feel fatigue until after they ran at top speeds for long distances in record times.

Remember, your body is extremely flexible and adjusts to the demands made on it. For example, if you stay in bed for a week, you'll find that your muscles, heart, lungs, and circulation quickly adapt. Their efficiency will decrease drastically because they don't need to be particularly efficient. Even your bone marrow will stop producing so many red blood cells because fewer are being destroyed by activity.

The point is, unlike many other sophisticated machines, the human body improves with use. So for an investment in your future well-being, find some time to exercise regularly. The typical Masters athlete does this. He is between fifty and ninety years old and usually began serious training about twenty years earlier. Drs. Shephard and Kavanagh said, "The majority of the competitors tested were average rather than outstanding, achieving between 80 percent and 90 percent of record speeds [in running]. The older competitors over short and medium distances attained only 60 percent to 80 percent of world records for their class." These Masters ran an average of thirty-five miles a week.

"Many of the athletes were taking dietary supplements," said the researchers. "The practice was particularly common among those in middle- and long-distance events. The items taken included megadoses of vitamin C, vitamin B mixtures, wheat germ oil, yogurt, vitamin E, and yeast extract. A number of the English competitors had also adopted a vegetarian diet." We will discuss dietary intake that goes along with rebounding aerobics in the final chapter of this book.

These Master runners had lower than the "normal" age-related resting blood pressures and pulse rates. There is clear evidence that regular endurance training can lower systemic blood pressures.

Their heart volumes, the amount of blood pumped around the body with each stroke of the heart muscle, was greater than those of sedentary adults. Twelve of the 135 contestants measured had volumes of more than 14 ml/kg, compared with 10 ml/kg in a sedentary man. Furthermore, group averages were not only maintained but even increased as the contestants became older.

In conclusion, Shephard and Kavanagh wrote: "In general, the Masters athlete is more fit than his contemporaries in the general population. He shows a lesser accumulation of subcutaneous fat, a better preservation of lean tissue, a lower resting blood pressure, a greater work performance at a given target heart rate, a slower aging of aerobic power, a larger heart volume, and a lesser likelihood of ST segment abnormalities at a given heart rate. All of these advantages are known responses to regular long, slow distance training."[5]

Rebounding Turns Back the Years

Elva and Theodore "Ted" Jodar of Edmonds, Washington are Masters Athletes in their own right. They perform the regular long training procedures for themselves in two ways. They have won several awards as experts in ballroom dancing and square dancing, and they do a morning set of rebounding exercises to get themselves going. Elva, age sixty-three and four feet, nine inches tall, weighing in at less than 100 pounds, and Ted, age seventy-seven, five feet, four inches tall, weighing 115 pounds, rebound immediately upon arising. They adhere to the admonition to "shake well before using."

Ted said, "I never rebound less than ten minutes and usually about fifteen minutes."

Elva said, "I bounce to music because I love to dance. And I rebound at least a half hour but not as vigorously as does Ted. He does it the doctor way, but I just have fun."

Ted said, "I do my rebounding according to the location of the various organs in the body. I attempt to strengthen each one as I'm moving. I don't just jump up and down for fun. I use the pressure points of the body with my fingers. As I am rebounding I place the tips of my fingers into the main organ points, probing and palpating here and there as I'm moving. If I find any spots that are tender, I concentrate on those spots

[5]Roy J. Shephard and Terence Kavanagh. "The effects of training on the aging process." *The Physician and Sports Medicine,* January 1978, pp. 33-40.

with pressure applied while I bounce. If you have any sore spots, you can get rid of them with fingertip pressure while rebounding just like that. It's very simple. This procedure tends to concentrate your thoughts and inner energy right at the tenderness. By directing your own innate, inborne energy to that spot for correction and making it strong, you'll accomplish some healing for yourself."

Elva said, "You might call it **visualization.** You visualize whatever health problem you might have to help as being very good, healthy and whole. And then it becomes healed faster by rebounding because your body will direct your thought energies to make itself well."

Ted said, "At our age, we do not believe in taking drugs — poisons — to correct defects in the body. We use the more natural remedies where we can. This is something I learned at a very early age."

Elva said, "The body has the potential of healing itself. Given a chance with the proper exercise, food, and rest, it will do exactly that."

"Given time," Ted replied, "the body will manufacture an antidote against any poison. Rebounding exercise helps the body make such antidotes. Not only that, it furnishes you with more balance and coordination. Do you know when you can tell that a man is aged prematurely? When he has lost his ability to sustain balance — when he can't stand in the middle of the floor and put on a pair of pants. That's a good test.

"One more piece of advice I would give a senior citizen is that when he or she gets a rebounding device, start with it slow and easy. Don't use it more than two minutes at a time but use it ten times a day. You'll shake out the old toxins from your body systems," said Ted Jodar.

Dr. Herbert A. deVries, director of the exercise laboratory at the Andrus Gerontology Center at the University of Southern California in Los Angeles, says that exercise is certainly not the illusory fountain of youth, but it does help to turn back the years by increasing the heart's ability to pump blood. This pumping function declines about 8 percent each decade after adulthood. Blood pressure increases with age, as fatty deposits clog the arteries. By middle age, the opening of the coronary arteries is closed by 29 percent of what it was when you were in your twenties. As you get on in years, lung capacity decreases also and the chest wall stiffens, reducing the amount of oxygen available to your body tissues. The skeletal muscles gradually lose strength, and endurance for muscular activity is reduced.

Your body's capacity to accomplish work, as measured by the maximum of oxygen it can use, has reduced by age seventy-five to less than half what it was at age twenty. Reaction time and speed of movement slow, as nerve cells age. Bones gradually lose minerals, soften and shrink, and fracture easily. With the passage of each decade, three to five percent of muscle tissue is actually lost. At the same time, the percentage of your body that is fat increases. To retain the same proportion of fat to lean body mass, you have to weigh less and less as you get older.

"So many people rust out before they wear out because they fail to realize that the human body was made to be used for as long as a person lives," says Dr. Robert E. Wear, exercise physiologist at the University of New Hampshire.

But research conducted by Dr. Everett L. Smith at the University of Wisconsin among persons who average eighty-four years of age showed that exercise can halt body deterioration. It can even halt the loss of bone and increase the size of bones, thereby strengthening them. The more that nerve cells are used, the less likely they are to age.

Exercise prevents joints from wearing out. Elderly people who move their joints in routine fitness programs were found to have less arthritic changes in their hips than older sedentary folk.

When the aged exercise, says Dr. Wear, who has developed exercise programs for people in nursing homes, "their appearance improves, they feel better, their energy reserves increase, they eat better, their peripheral circulation improves, and their range of motion increases. There's a tremendous difference in their vigor and vitality, and they're much less likely to suffer the catastrophic falls that old people are prone to."[6]

Lewis Cains, President of Enhancement Products International Corporation of Thousand Oaks, California, dispenses rebound units in nursing homes. Cains says, "I have been turning vegetables into human beings. I interest the most forceful old person in the nursing home, the ring leader, so-to-speak, in trying out the rebounding device. He or she gets on it to bounce a little bit. I go away leaving behind this rebound unit, and when I return I usually find the whole place is bouncing. Elderly people who were formerly afraid to even get up and walk around become active again. They bounce away, play chess and checkers, talk to each other, and renew their interest in living again. Rebounding does this for the elderly.

"I have to warn the user though that you can't bounce to a dead room. You have to listen to sound! Listen to music or a cassette teaching tape, talk on the telephone, carry on a conversation with others in the room, or listen to something else like that; otherwise bouncing for ten minutes without diversion will have you feeling bored," assured Cains.

The need to keep yourself young and vital as years advance is a necessary requisite for all Americans. The fastest-growing segments of the United States elderly population over the next half-century will be the very old, according to an April 1978 Government study.

The report by the Department of Human Services'

---

[6]Jane E. Brody. "Exercising to turn back the years." *The New York Times,* June 6, 1979, P. C18 and C19.

Office of Human Development noted that the population sixty and older has soared from 4.9 million in 1900 to nearly 33 million in 1977, and is expected to hit 71 million by 2035.

The nation's total population, 76 million in 1900 and now 220 million, is expected to grow only 40 percent to 304 million by 2035. "While the size of the population sixty and over has increased by nearly seven times since 1900, the population seventy-five and over has experienced a tenfold increase and the eighty-five-plus age group has grown by about seventeen times," the report said. By 2035, one-third of the elderly will be over seventy-five and one-tenth over eighty-five.

"White female children now can expect to live to seventy-five, or eight years longer than white males."[7]

Keeping these facts in mind, the way to survive for the next fifty-five years is to keep fit and avoid senility with rebounding aerobics.

Such an aerobic exercise is one of the main methods of retaining cognitive performance with age, as recommended in a newly published book co-authored by Abram Hoffer, M.D., Ph. D. and Morton Walker, D.P.M., *Nutrients to Age Without Senility.*[8] Those who are old already, those who refuse to accept the concept that any aging takes place at all, and those of us who appear to be growing older are quite aware of the potential of senility. We see it around us; read of the myriad numbers wasting their minds doing nothing after retirement; witness it among older loved ones, neighbors, and friends. Senility is sad to see come upon formerly alert and active performers on the stage of life.

Exercise physiologists have looked at biological measures demonstrating the benefit of leading a physically active life. Psychologists, in describing psychological changes with increased age, have examined a

---

[7] "Old-Age Trends Cited." *The New York Times,* April 12, 1978, p. 32.

[8] Abram Hoffer and Morton Walker. *Nutrients to Age without Senility.* (New Canaan, Connecticut: Keats Publishing, Inc., 1980), pp. 189-199.

broad range of variables. The cognitive performance decrements in aging seem to be the criterior by which scientists measure whether or not an elderly person is senile.[9]

Senility is defined as physical or mental deterioration that occurs in some persons in their later years. It is most often applied to the mental and emotional difficulties that sometimes appear in the elderly such as extreme irritability, anxiety, loss of memory, depression, and a loss of ability to maintain proper feeding and dressing habits. In its most extreme form, senility is sometimes referred to as senile dementia or psychosis; the person may need constant supervision and treatment.

Cognitive performance is general terminology referring to the quality of knowing what is happening around you. It includes perceiving, recognizing, conceiving, judging, sensing, reasoning, and imagining and acting on these aspects of thinking and planning.

Cognitive performance may be affected by changes in the brain, or it may not. In many cases of senility, no sign can be found of significant brain changes. The elderly person just begins to feel useless because, with advancing age, he or she is denied any meaningful role in society. This is a crime our society commits on the older, formerly productive population.

Frustration builds upon frustration, until there is a withdrawal from life and regression to infantile behavior. This kind of senility can definitely be prevented, or its effects can be minimized, by involving older people in programs of fitness or other rewarding activities that give them a sense of worth. Rebounding fills part of this need exceedingly well. It's something any older individual can do for himself, privately or among friends to avoid lapsing into the worthless feelings that bring on senility.

---

[9]D. Arenberg. "Cognition and aging: verbal learning, memory problems solving and aging." *The Psychology of Adult Development and Aging.* eds. C. Eisdorfer and M. Lawton: (Washington, D.C.: American Psychological Association, 1973), pp. 74-97.

Cognitive performance loss with aging has been related to the progressive degeneration of the central nervous system (CNS) via the biological aging process.[10],[11] It's also tied to cardiovascular or cerebrovascular disease.[12],[13] Both of these deteriorations in the body may be avoided, however, by your influencing your cardiorespiratory health by leading a physically active life. You can retain your cognitive performance this way as you grow older.

As you age, for a variety of reasons the blood supply to the CNS becomes less efficient, thereby causing slowing of brain functions. Animal studies have supported this position and indicate that motor neurons can adapt to increases in physiological strain through exercise by enhancing their oxidative enzyme activity as does skeletal muscle.[14] In addition, researchers have found that exercised rats had positive changes on the structure and function of the nervous system.[15]

In determining your own potential for senility, measure as the medical scientists and gerontologists do; they check the patients reaction time (RT). This is done for several reasons. First of all, RT provides an excellent indication of how effectively and efficiently the pro-

[10]J.E. Birren. "Translations in gerontology — from lab to life: psychophysiology and the speed of response." *American Psychology* 29:808-815, 1974.

[11]J.E. Birren and W. Spieth. "Age, response speed, and cardiovascular functions. *Journal of Gerontology* 17:390-391, 1962.

[12]W. Speith. "Slowness of task performance and cardiovascular diseases." *Behavior. Aging. and the Nervous System,* eds. A.T. Welford and J.E. Birren. (Springfield, Ill.: Charles C. Thomas, 1965), pp. 366-400.

[13]G.E. Talland, "Initiation of response and reaction time in aging and brain damage." *Behavior. Aging. and the Nervous System,* eds. A.T. Welford and J.E. Birren. (Springfield, Illinois: Charles C. Thomas, 1965), pp. 526-561.

[14]L. Gerchman, V. Edgerton, and R. Carrow. "Effects of physical training on histochemistry and morphology of ventral motor neurons." *Experimental Neurology* 49:790-901, 1975.

[15]E. Retzlaff and J. Fontaine. "Functional and structural changes in motor neurons with age. *Behavior. Aging. and the Nervous System,* eds. A.T. Welford and J.E. Birren. (Springfield, Ill.: Charles C. Thomas, 1965), pp. 340-352.

cesses of the CNS are working.[16] Reaction time is a predictor of senility, since it slows with age, and any mediating effect due to poor cardiovascular health shows up as marked reduction in the usual age-RT.[17,18] It is directly related to cardiovascular disease.[19, 20, 21] Our advice to you is to keep up your cardiovascular fitness as we described in chapter two by engaging in rebounding aerobics. It's the means to avoiding senility.

[16]R. Marteniuk. *Information Processing in Motor Skills.* (New York: Holt, Rinehart, and Winston, 1976), pp. 106-122.

[17]S. Ferris, F. Crook, G. Sathananthan, and S. Gershan. "Reaction as a diagnostic measure in senility."*J. American Geriatric Society* 24:543-548, 1974.

[18]G.E. Talland, *Op. cit.*

[19]J. Abrahams and J. Birren. "Reaction time as a function of age and behavior predisposition to coronory heart disease."*Journal of Gerontology* 28:471-478, 1973.

[20]W. Speith, *Op. cit.*

[21] J.E. Birren and W. Speith, *Op. cit.*

7

Human Physiologic Functioning in Reboundology

During eight years of marriage, Mrs. Laverne Groff of Stevens, Pennsylvania, age twenty-eight, had been in and out of hospitals more often than anyone should be subjected to such medical attention. She was a very sick woman.

"I had one operation after another," she wrote us for publication. "The first year Paul and I were married I had my first surgery for an ovary that had ruptured. After the operation the doctor told me that I should thank the Dear Lord every day to be alive, because I had hemorrhaged on the table. My doctor said that in one more minute the blood would have gone over my heart.

"The gynecological surgeon had taken out one half of the ruptured ovary and patched up the remaining part. But in less than a year the same thing happened to the other half — a rupture — so I went through it all over again.

"In a little over six months my other ovary did the same thing," continued Mrs. Groff. "This time my heart stopped when I was in the recovery room following the third surgery. The doctor really worked at me and got my heart going again in a short time. While recuperating from this latest procedure, I was still as sick and full of pain as before the operation. Consequently, the physicians put me under some more testing and found something else wrong. It was not a week yet since I had undergone the last operation when the surgeon said to me that he was so very sorry, but I must go right to the operating room for still a fourth procedure.

"I cried out, 'Oh, No! It just cannot be me again.' But it sure was me, and my body had no time at all to get built up. It was just too much. In a short time following the latest operation my body gave out entirely so that my muscles and nerves went haywire. I was struck by a strange muscle condition where I couldn't talk for over two months. I couldn't eat by myself. I seemed to have lost all strength. That means I was unable to raise my arms up and down, and walking was absolutely out for me," explained the woman.

"After I finally left the hospital I still had so much pain because of a very bad back problem. These operations seemed to have messed up my back completely. This is when I began to get help from a chiropractor. I really did get relief with chiropractic treatment, but my back was soon out of place again and my muscles would be hurting terribly. Therefore, I was still looking for something else to help me," she acknowledged.

"My husband and I attended one of Dr. C. Samuel West's self-help clinics, and we realized that we just had to learn more about how to help me in the future. Dr. West taught us how I should sit in a chair with my feet on the rebounding unit while my husband stood on it and bounced my legs up and down. We worked together this way for a few minutes and did it quite often each day. In several weeks, I was able to get on the unit myself. And in a couple of months I was feeling so much strength coming into my body. I could just feel my insides getting stronger, and the chiropractor and my family physician both commented on the big change they saw in me. My family doctor said that if he hadn't seen my condition before and witnessed my improvement with his own eyes, he wouldn't have believed I was the same person.

"Then the most wonderful thing occurred; I became pregnant with our first baby. The doctor said that if I hadn't acquired so much strength in my insides I could never be carrying a child almost nine months. He was born weighing six pounds thirteen and a half ounces and was twenty inches in length. Isn't that amazing that I became pregnant with just half an ovary intact?

"We moved into our new house and have been enjoying our little Brian Lee ever so much," said the new mother. "At the time of this writing our baby is four and a half months old and fifteen pounds. Ever since coming home from the hospital, I've been doing all my housework and taking care of our child. I attribute my recovery to being taught how to use the rebounding unit correctly so my body could heal itself."

Could the rebounding device and instruction on how to use lymphatic exercises be responsible for restoration of physiological functioning to this woman who had been so beset by gynecological and muscular weaknesses? Could instituting *reboundology be the source of adequate ovarian performance so that even with just 25 percent of her ovary capacity intact, Mrs. Groff still became pregnant and carried the baby almost full term? The answer to both questions is a qualified "yes."

Most likely, Mrs. Laverne Groff had a full body cell response to changes in gravity. She experienced human physiologic refunctioning in *reboundology. All of her recuperative powers were concentrated into self-healing by the mechanisms of rebounding aerobics.

Research by Albert E. Carter, President of the National Institute of Reboundology and Health, Inc. in Edmonds, Washington, indicates that alterations in the gravitational pull of the earth cause a direct reponse

*See pg. iii

from the cells of your body.

From his literature search, Al Carter learned of the automatic adjustment of cells to their own environment; any change tends to cause a cellular reaction. The cell gets stronger from mechanical stimulation supplied by the gravitational pull. Rebounding produces a continuous cellular response because of constant changes in gravity while in vertical motion.

Carter says, "Rebound exercise is a method of stimulating every cell of the body simultaneously by increasing the G force applied to every cell. We do that by vertically adding the forces of acceleration and deceleration to the ever-present gravitational pull. Every cell in the body then begins to automatically adjust to the new environment."[1]

Thus, the G force at the top of the bounce is eliminated and the body becomes weightless for a fraction of a second. At the bottom of the bounce when you touch the mat the G force suddenly doubles over what is ordinary gravity on earth and internal organs are put under pressure. Their cellular stimulation is increased accordingly so that waste materials within cells get squeezed out. The lymphatics carry the waste away to be disposed of through the urinary and other excretory mechanisms. Rebounding makes the body cleaner.

The increased G force also puts cell walls under stress causing them to undergo an individual training effect. The aerobics of rebounding brings more oxygen for penetration by osmosis from the blood. Each cell gets the amount of nourishment it requires on which to thrive.

This combination of excretion of wastes and incorporation of nourishment, both done more efficiently than any ordinary program of exercise, conditions the cells beyond their usual threshold. They get stronger

[1]Albert E. Carter. *The Miracles of Rebound Exercise*. (Snohomish, Washington: The National Institute of Reboundology and Health, 1979), p. 80.

and gain endurance to cope better with the stresses encountered in daily life.

This probably happened to the cells in Laverne Groff's body, especially to her remaining one-half ovary. And although she has repeated her story here after having told it in *Miracles of Rebound Exercise,* her case history is illustrative of what can occur when the science of rebounding is applied to a potential medical catastrophe.[2]

Optimal Physical Functioning by Rebounding

A great deal of attention and discussion has been given by exercise physiologists, laypersons anxious to adopt a holistic lifestyle, doctors reacting to the public's demands to be taught about their bodies, medical journalists, health educators, and others to the ill-defined concept called "physical fitness." This is an all-encompassing term used to indicate physiologic readiness for any type of physical activity. It has been applied to advertise electric-powered exercise bicycles, jogging, isometric ropes, honey, bread, milk, high protein drinks, and even rebounding devices.

Seldom is the term applied to the natural optimal physical functioning by the organs, tissues, and cells of the body — to their individual performance capacity. Nevertheless, "physical fitness" actually refers to the ability of certain body systems and, therefore, the total human organism to perform. This is the true meaning of the term. And, Mrs. Groff is an example of physical fitness applied in its correct sense. From having almost no physical functioning of her ovaries — in fact, from a state of malfunctioning — her ovarian tissue that was left produced the egg that birthed a healthy baby boy of almost seven pounds.

The women's ovarian refunctioning most likely took place from rebounding aerobics as one of several fac-

[2]*Ibid.* pp. 157 & 158.

tors involved with her recovery. The importance no doubt of each of the other factors were specific to the organ and its activity, as well. Human physiological functioning is dependent on seven particular elements, and the following listing is presented as a way to categorize these elements:

1) Energy release processes — the aerobic and anaerobic metabolic processes (involving oxygen and not involving oxygen).

2) Energy sources available — the availability of food stuffs or substrates that contain potential energy.

3) Nutrient resources — the coenzymes and other factors that synergize or catalyze the chemical reactions within the body.

4) Genetic makeup — the inherited characteristics not only of external features, personality quirks, and intelligence, but also the strengths and weaknesses of the interior environment of the body.

5) Psychological attitude and emotional involvement.

6) The environment — ecologic alterations that cause the body to react to ambient conditions (such as allergy).

7) The oxygen supply — delivery of an abundant consumption capacity.

These seven factors and more came together for Mrs. Groff, perhaps stimulated by lessons in the use of the rebound exercise unit. They assisted the woman into an optimal state of physical functioning. At the very least, rebound exercise was the key that excited Mrs. Groff into taking hold of her own health situation and applying her personal power of self-healing. In doing this, she instituted a number of different performance requirements on her internal organs and muscles. She subjected them to demands for individual performance capacities, and the organs delivered.

We will now discuss the separate physiological reasons why human work performance and human cellular enhancement take place in the body. You'll learn why *reboundology helps the body to heal itself.

*See pg. iii

In Harmony with the "On-Off" Impulse of the Universe

The rebounding mechanism brings about a number of vague and difficult to explain mental and physical responses that are tied to the laws of physics. We'll present these effects first and then move on to the more tangible biological basis for the enhancement of functional capacity by each body organ.

The gentle bounce exercise of rebounding has been exceedingly effective in returning natural, regular bowel movements to chronically constipated individuals. This is documented in case histories and in anecdotes related by the patients, themselves. The steady bounce sets up a pulsating rhythm transmitted by the nervous system to the vital hindbrain mechanism which regulates the functioning of the intestinal system. This pulsation seems to serve as a catalyst to the reestablishment of rhythmical bowel activity. Digestion improves, in general.

The autonomic nervous system falls into a sine wave activity of "on-off, on-off," which is the three dimensional wave motion of the entire physical universe at all levels. The "on-off" is responsible for the physiological conduction of nervous impulses along a neuron. Nervous activity of the bowel creates muscular activity, and normal bowel function becomes restored. By supplying this gentle, regular pattern of pulsation with rebounding, a person places himself in harmony with the "on-off" impulse of the universe and gets a beneficial physiological result.

The most obvious benefit for a constipated person is restoration of natural movement of the bowel. At the level of the brain, however, the pulsing activity can and does bring about bilateral coordination of the cerebral hemispheres. As one bounces, neural impulses are set up along both limbs. Simultaneously and equally, those impulses cross over at the hindbrain but remain equal in strength. When they are perceived at the cortical hemispheres, the pulses are able to be seen on an electroencephalogram. They are visualized as coordinated, synchronized, coherent brain wave activity. This indicates there is a greater level of mental activity scientists have labelled "the eureka experience."

There are parallels to this eureka experience in studies done with Transcendental Meditation and in studies performed to investigate genius problem solving. The eureka experience has been noted by psychiatrists who have studied problem solving activity of the mind. When a problem solver has the sudden insight into a perplexing problem ("Eureka") and finds the solution, a distinct pattern of brain activity takes place. Brainwaves cross cortical hemispheres and something unique physiologically accompanies the mental or eureka experience. Rebounding does this. It brings on the eureka experience similar to the mental accuity often present when a meditator comes out of his deeper level of mind.

Since all of the universe is made up of energy in the form of light (quantum theory) or wave motion or particle motion, it is recognized there is alternation of activity and rest at the finest level. This is "on-off" activity and is fundamental to the maintenance of the physical universe. Its regularity brings about stability.

While bounding on the rebound unit, you feel a complete absence of the concept of time. You move into a higher state of consciousness. There is a sense of restful alert activity of the mind that is calming and spiritual. It is a re-experiencing of the gentle knee bounce in babyhood we had received from mother.

If you perform certain physiological tests on yourself while engaging in rebounding aerobics, you'll find a series of changes are taking place. For example, oxygen consumption and metabolic rate increase; breath rate increases; the depth of inspiration increases; skin resistance increases, indicating a reduction of anxiety or emotional disturbances (contrary to stress situations where skin resistance decreases); the cardiac output increases by means of a stronger blood surge with each beat; the work load of the heart reduces; the concentration of blood level of lactate decreases, indicating no fatigue despite muscle movement; mental reaction time speeds up, indicating increased alertness, improved coordination of mind and body, reduced dullness, and improved efficiency in perception and performance.

There are changes in your brain wave pattern, while bouncing, showing a spread of eight to nine cycles per second waves to the more frontal areas of the brain with the occasional occurrence of prominent and synchronized five to seven cycles per second waves. These patterns are different from those seen in other states of consciousness and mean that while you are rebounding you are in a state of restful inner alertness.

Furthermore, you experience increased perceptual ability with an improvement of hearing and increased clarity and refinement of perception during the movements and afterward.

You feel increased stability and have fewer spontaneous galvanic skin responses. Rebounding aerobics stabilizes the nervous system, and this stabilization continues to maintain itself after you step off the rebound exercise unit. The consequence is that you have more resistance to environmental, physical and mental stress. You won't develop psychosomatic disease or behavioral instability, and there is greater efficiency in the activity of your nervous system which provides you with more energy for purposeful activity. All this is proven by means of the galvanic skin response test to a stressful stimulus. The smoother graph of a person who rebounds regularly indicates a more stable functioning of his nervous system, allowing him to interact more effectively with his environment.

Indeed, by doing rebounding aerobics daily, you perform faster and more accurately in complex perceptual motor situations. You'll have greater coordination between the mind and body, increased perceptual awareness, neuromuscular integration, and feel greater flexibility in your thinking. Individual studies show that rebounding people perform better on recall tests and learn more quickly than others, especially after they come off the rebounding apparatus. They show significantly better results on more difficult puzzles, possibly because of improved memory and learning ability.

Finally, rebounding aerobics offers spiritual inspiration and peace of mind with the universe. You will notice a reduction in your nervousness, aggression, emotional instability, self-criticism and self-doubt, inhibition, irritability, and depression.

You'll witness an increase in your sense of freedom, self-assuredness and self-confidence, good humor, positive thinking, staying power and efficiency, sociability, liveliness, tolerance in frustrating situations, harmony with others, respect for others, cordiality, friendliness, effectiveness in persuading others, and an inner contentment.

For those who must confront their addiction to tranquilizers, stimulants, and other drugs, rebounding aerobics provides part of the antidote to removing them from one's lifestyle. It does this by improving the sense of well-being, strengthening mental health and thereby directly removing the need for drugs.

Respiration in Reboundology

Pulmonary ventilation increases rapidly after the beginning of rebounding and reaches a plateau which is determined by the height, the speed, the force, and the relative amount of the bounce. Arterial blood lactate concentration is not the cause of this increased oxygen uptake as it is with other forms of exercise. The higher ventilation is augmented by a rise in both the amount of air sucked in with each inhalation and the breathing frequency. Bouncing brings on greater pulmonary action.

This is one of the reasons that rebounding exercises may help tobacco and marijuana addicts to cut down on their smoking. There is an increased aerobic metabolism during the exercises with increased ventilation and gas exchange in the lungs becoming necessary. Adequate alveolar ventilation, sufficient numbers of red blood cells in the pulmonary capillaries, and normal ratios between ventilation and perfusion are factors of importance. The large ventilation during rebounding leads to a considerable increase in the energy expenditure of the respiratory muscles and respiration will become a limiting factor for smokers.

Unless they are absolutely intent in pursuing their death wish, which makes them blind to their reduced ventilation capacity, the smokers will recognize their need to take in more oxygen per liter of air consumption. Tidal volume increases in both the inspiratory and expiratory direction during rebounding aerobics. But a smoker will have so damaged his alveoli (while he continues as a persistent smoker), he won't be able to utilize the required oxygen. This is because the total ventilation is divided into the ventilation of "dead space" and that of the alveoli.

At a given total ventilation, a higher breathing rate as is necessary in rebounding, is concomitant with lower alveolar ventilation. There is a tendency of the "physiological dead space" to increase with smoking. The alveolar ventilation increases from 70 percent of the total pulmonary ventilation at rest to about 90 percent of total ventilation during rebounding. If physiological dead space has been pathologically created from smoking, the smoker will realize an inadequate alveolar expansion. Simply, he won't perform well at all on the rebound unit. Thus, rebounding is a test of the extent of damage a smoker inflicts on his ability to breathe and extract oxygen from the air.

While performing rebounding aerobics, the forces against which the respiratory muscles have to work are: (1) elastic forces in the tissues of the lung and chest wall, (2) flow-resistive forces in the airways and tissues, and (3) inertial forces which depend upon the mass of the gas and the tissues. The work done against inertia is negligible. At rest most of the respiratory work is done against elastic forces. With increasing ventilation during rebounding, the flow-resistive work rises rapidly.[3]

The oxygen cost of breathing for the same ventilation is about 40 percent higher when you rebound than when you sit in a comfortable chair.[4] At a ventilation of sixty liters per minute (l/min), 4 percent of the total energy you expend is used for breathing. During a vigorous bouncing session with ventilations of 110 to 120 l/min the corresponding value rises to at least 9 percent. That's the amount of energy you use just to breathe.

Pursuing the highest and most rapid bounce for a prolonged period on your rebounding device, the maximal possible ventilation you could expend would be between 130 and 170 l/min.[5] The work of breathing is not a limiting factor for rebounding under other than extreme conditions such as performing at a high altitude or inhaling the smoke of perhaps sixty cigarettes a day.

Blood Circulation in *Reboundology

How is oxygen transport to working muscles increased in response to the challenge of mild to maximal rebounding aerobics? How is oxygen transport maintained when rebounding is prolonged and demands on the cardiovascular system for heat transport from the muscles are gradually superimposed? These are questions which might be considered when the purchaser of a rebound unit compares his new exercising device to the competition of other ways to exercise.

---

[3]A.B. Otis. "The work of breathing." In *Handbook of Physiology*, section 3, vol. I: 463-476, Washington, D.C., 1964.

[4]M. Nielsen. "Sie respirationsarbeit bei korperuhe and bei muskelarbeit." *Skand. Arch. Physiol.* 74:299-316, 1936.

[5]R. Margaria, J. Milic-Emili, J.M. Petit, and G. Cavagna. "Mechanical work of breathing during muscular exercise."*J. Appl. Physiol.* 15:354-358, 1960.

*See pg. iii

In chapter eleven we will focus on the advantages and disadvantages of jogging and running. Here we'll examine responses to graded intensities of exercise in general.

Once oxygen is absorbed into the red blood cells in the pulmonary circulation, the transport to working muscles is increased by increasing cardiac output and arterio-venous (a-v) oxygen difference. The circulatory response to rebounding is a function of age, sex, posture, and the muscle mass of an individual. The a-v maximum oxygen extraction to nourish the muscle cells is 85 to 90 percent. That's the most oxygen you can get from your blood with the greatest exercise effort, for any exercise movement. This is the exact amount of oxygen extraction achieved with forty minutes of rebounding aerobics performed at the fastest speed by an athlete with very high maximal oxygen uptake (VO_2).[6]

Heat transport from the moving muscles is maintained by sacrificing the blood flow to the splanchnic region of the body. The splanchnic takes in the viscera or gut comprising the contents of the abdominal cavity. The splanchnic region normally receives 20 to 25 percent of the total cardiac output at rest, but during exercise the blood flow is shunted away from this area. Up to 400 milliliters of oxygen per minute can be redistributed from the splanchnic region to actively working muscle without any additional increase in cardiac output.[7] This is a main reason why you should not ingest food before engaging in rebounding aerobics. There is very little blood flow to nourish the organs of digestion and even less to assist in the process of absorption.

Moreover, blood flow to the skin, as with visceral organs, may be progressively comprised with increasing demands for oxygen transport to the muscles. A person

[6]L.B. Rowell, J.R. Blackmon, and R.A. Bruce. "Indocyanine green clearance and estimated hepatic blood flow during mild to maximal exercise in upright man." *J. Clin. Investigation* 43:1677-1690, 1964.

[7]*Ibid.*

with a weak heart will actually stop the skin blood flow in an effort to supply sufficient blood flow to actively working muscles.

In comparison with other exercises that have a person planting his feet on the ground (except swimming), rebounding aerobics provides a more favorable advantage to the exerciser. That is, the effects of gravity are eliminated and central circulatory changes are less.[8]

Energy Release in Rebounding Muscles

Skeletal muscle, in addition to having the basic properties common to all tissue, possesses the ability to contract and move the body. This contraction, however, requires that a large amount of energy be released. In fact, the metabolic rate of skeletal muscle can increase more than any other tissue of the body. Thus, while the skeletal muscles consume a small percent of the oxygen uptake at rest, during heavy rebounding, when the total body metabolic rate is increased fifteen to twenty times that of rest, most of this increase occurs in the working muscles where the metabolic rate may be as much as 100 times higher than at rest.

The energy needed for rebounding aerobics is derived from oxidation of carbohydrates and fat and from splitting of glycogen and energy-rich phosphates in the muscle cells. During prolonged rebounding of ten minutes or more, the energy needed comes from fats and carbohydrates as the major fuels consumed. Protein degradation occurs only under fasting conditions when the reserves of fat and carbohydrates have been significantly depleted. During short exhaustive work periods on the rebounding device for a person out of shape, the energy needed comes mostly from glycogen and phosphates.

When your muscles contract during rebounding, the

[8]L.B. Rowell, J.A. Murray, G.L. Brengelmann, and K.K. Kraning II. "Human cardiovascular adjustments to rapid changes in skin temperature during exercise." *Circulatory Research*, March 1970, pp. 131-137.

cleavage of adenosine triphosphate (ATP) provides the energy for the contraction of your skeletal muscles. In order to maintain the process of contraction it is, therefore, necessary to provide a continuous supply of ATP. This is done through taking in the best possible nutrition, and by continuing your training program as much as you can. Studies on animals have shown that the stores of ATP and an associated enzyme called phosphocreatine are increased during a training period.[9]

We have presented a series of physiological facts relating to rebounding aerobics which are highly technical and might be considered impractical in a book for popular distribution such as this one. Yet, there is much more to present. We've merely scratched the surface of the physiological effects of physical conditioning by rebounding. We hope to stimulate research by the rebound exercise industry through our presentation in this chapter of human physiological concepts of *reboundology.

Some of our technical information may be put into perspective when you consider the response of the human organism to exercising on the rebounder. The story of Mrs. Laverne Groff, cited at the beginning of this chapter, is an example. Or, evaluate the case history described to us by Mrs. Sara Glick of Lancaster, Pennsylvania. Mrs. Glick is an Amish lady who practices reflexology and attempts to bring about healing through the skill of her hands on the bottom of people's feet. Lately, she has added the rebound unit as one of the healing aides she teaches people to use. This came about as a result of a dramatic occurrence that took place in her own family.

Mrs. Glick's grandchild, Maryanne Fischer, age eight, who lives in Clinton County, Pennsylvania, became sick one morning. "She was tight in the chest," said Mrs. Glick. "She had a cough. We first gave her a

---

[9]A. Szent-Gyorgyi. *Chemistry of Muscular Contraction.* (New York: Academic Press, 1953).

*See page iii

natural remedy to try to get the mucous loose, but her chest continued to get tighter until she lapsed into semi-consciousness. Maryanne could hardly breathe.

"We attempted to reach a doctor, but none was available. So we had to look for something to do to give relief to this child. Her body temperature was beginning to rise. We set her to bouncing on the rebounding device and kept it up for forty-five minutes. My two youngest daughters and I took turns supporting the child on the unit. The mucous in her chest broke up on its own, and the child got to breathing better. She began to talk where she couldn't have spoken a word before the bouncing," said the grandmother. "The cold broke loose some more from more rebounding, and the child sweated tremendously. Her fever dropped and came right down to normal. The vibration caused her to spit up mucous something awful, but the bouncing really did it for Maryanne. She went to school the next day. It saved her from pneumonia and sold me on the merits of rebounding."

This is another practical illustration from everyday experience of human physiologic functioning coming out of *reboundology.

Remember! For optimal exercise effect, jump for health.

---

*See page iii

8

Coordination and Correction for the Learning Disabled Child

Camille Weicker of Washington, D.C., former wife of the United States Senator for Connecticut Lowell P. Weicker, Jr., had a premonition something was wrong when their son was born a little over ten years ago. She was correct.

The pediatrician said, "We're going to make some tests. Then we can tell you for sure."

But the head of the hospital genetics department arrived and said, "Camille, there's no sense in waiting and in giving you false hope. Your child has Downs' Syndrome."

"I didn't know what Down's Syndrome was. I only knew there was something wrong with my child," said Mrs. Weicker. Then the doctors told her the condition used to be called "Mongolism."

Children with Down's Syndrome — which occurs once in 600 to 1,000 live births — have an additional chromosome which results in mental retardation. Research shows that the older the mothers, the greater the risk, which increases dramatically over age thirty-five.[1]

Down's Syndrome is one of the more serious forms of learning and behavioral disorder collected under the single terminology of **minimal brain dysfunction.** At the last count there were about 100 different diagnoses for this variety of disorders lumped under the minimal brain dysfunction heading. Parents who have been forced to seek help for their children from a succession of psychiatrists are confused by the numerous dysfunctional descriptions such as autistic, hyperactive, hyperkinetic, learning disabled, minimally brain damaged, dyslexic, and the latest which is "Attention Deficit Disorder". Often there is little logical relationship between the different diagnoses.

D.M. Vuckovich, M.D., Head of Child Neurology, Professor of Neurology and Pediatrics, and Chairman of Neurology and Psychiatry, Columbus-Cuneo-Cabrini Medical Center and Loyola University of Chicago Stritch School of Medicine, Maywood, Illinois, observed that the term minimal brain dysfunction (MBD) seemed inappropriate in terms of "the neurological deficits and learning obdurations, which ultimately may lead to lowered self-esteem, poor capacity to relate to environment, and diminished motivational force. MBD cannot be considered 'minimal' in a child of average or superior intelligence who never reaches the academic and socio-economic goals of which he is capable. This lack of fulfillment is a disappointment to family, friends, teachers, and most important, to the child himself."

Dr. Vuckovich explained that MBD signifies a syndrome phenomenon which encompasses neurological, emotional, social, behavioral, and cognitive disorders of varied causes, within the framework of a normal level of intelligence. An extreme expression of the poor social adjustment of such children and young adults may be

---

[1]Jane Anderson, "Retarded son 'total joy' for Weickers." *The Advocate,* April 14, 1980, p. 2.

seen in cases of juvenile and adult criminality, he stated in a symposium on "Learning and Behavioral Disorders with Neurological Implications," that we attended.

"Until a more satisfactory terminology is established," Dr. Vuckovich suggested that "LBD" be considered as an acceptable semantic umbrella instead of "MBD" to accommodate "the spectrum of interrelated yet diverse disorders for learning and behavioral disorders with or without psychiatric and/or neurological impairment."

Thus, Dr. Vuckovich provides us with yet another term, LBD, learning and behavioral disorders, making 101 ways to describe children who were formerly called "morons," "imbeciles," "idiots," and "retarded". Out of deference to the sensibilities of the parents, these children with learning disabilities are now given less frightening labels such as "slow learner," "emotionally handicapped," "intellectually deprived," and others. The diagnoses of psychiatrists more often reflect their own training and personal preferences rather than the illnesses of their young patients. While all the time the only thing the parents want is the means to correct this nightmare besetting their learning disabled child.

The Underlying Problem of Incoordination

More children than you might imagine are affected by learning disabilities.

Of third and fourth year students in Chicago public schools, 15 percent are underachievers; of these, half are learning disabled.

In the entire State of Minnesota, of students in kindergarten and grades one and two, 41 percent have learning problems; of these, one quarter require special placement services.

In St. Louis, 4 percent of all grade school children ages five to eleven have minimal brain dysfunction.

Ten percent of the second grade in Vermont schools suffer from learning problems.

In Guelph, Ontario, out of 1,307 pre-kindergarten children 16 percent were ill with a variety of emotional or behavioral difficulties.

The United States Office of Education estimates that 10 percent of the whole school population in the nation is ill mentally.

None of the percentages given here are guesses. They come directly from published investigations made by physicians researching in the educational field.

Of the best total estimate of learning and behavioral disorders, about 10 percent of all children born will have one or another of these 101 labelled conditions. That means that seven million Americans and seven hundred thousand Canadian families are affected directly. It is this 10 percent of our total number of families who will be vitally interested in the substance of this chapter which addresses itself to the underlying problem of incoordination and its correction for the learning disabled child.

In an exclusive interview, Alfhild Akselsen, Ph.D. of Beaumont, Texas, founder of the Texas Association of Children with Learning Disabilities of Austin, Texas, told us, "Learning disabled children have extremely poor coordination, balance, and rhythm. For correction, you have to trace the children's development back to where and when they deviated from normal, and start from there. Often the children lack physical strength, while others are enormously strong. However, the usual difficulty bringing on a lack of coordination is that one side of the body is not working. Also occurring might be that the left arm and right foot are very weak — problems on both sides — but most of the time the weakness is on one side that needs strengthening and rebuilding.

"A child might exhibit dysgraphia, an inability to write, or have mixed dominance. The child may be rightsided with a lot of difficulty using the right hand so that he or she switches to using the left hand and shows lefthandedness. Yet, when the child is corrected out of the problem, he or she may revert to being right-handed again, perhaps two years after complete developmental treatment began," Dr. Akselsen said.

The cause of this dysfunctioning of coordination between the body and brain are variable. Cigarette smoking by the mother during pregnancy may be the source of brain injury to her baby. The taking of any kind of drug, alcoholic beverage, environmental contamination, prolonged labor, or the administering of medication during the delivery are other causes. Certainly the "average American diet" of food additives, junk food, and highly processed food is a potential source of learning disability, even if the child escapes birth damage.

The greatest cause by far, however, is the preventing of a baby to creep and crawl and explore. Putting him or her in a playpen for safe-keeping interrupts the free flow of knowledge from integrating into the brain centers so that they will later function in patterns and give wrong perspectives to the youngster. Creeping and crawling, grasping and eyeing by the infant give him experience of his surroundings.

From the tonic neck reflex, where the baby feels the compulsion to turn his body in the direction in which the head is moved, the infant goes on to develop in his higher neurological and intellectual centers. Then he advances into the homolateral, or one-sided crawl. Lying on his stomach, he pushes with the hand and leg on the side to which his face was turned; then he turns his face and pushes with the other hand and leg. These movements are the beginning of coordination. Deny a baby his desire to creep and crawl, and you'll be planting the seeds of incoordination, lack of rhythm, and loss of balance that will show up in the near- or long-term.

The Symptoms of Minimal Brain Damage

When Peter Spiller of Millburn, New Jersey was eight years old he blurted out to his mother one day: "I wish I was in somebody else's body." Arlene Spiller asked him to explain. The child replied: "I wish I had somebody else's arms and legs and head." Peter's yearning touched his mother deeply, for the young man, now twenty-two, was a brain-injured child who cannot catch a ball, who is, in Mrs. Spiller's words, "clumsy and klutzy."

Because his learning skills are minute, Peter will lose the content of a conversation. He cannot hold onto "one thought after another, and another," his mother said. "Two minutes into a movie and he's lost the whole thing." Yet he reads and writes well and spells flawlessly.

Peter was erroneously diagnosed as mentally retarded at the age of eighteen months. "Go home and live with it," the pediatrician told the Spillers. They went, frantic, from doctor to doctor through conflicting opinions, until finally a neurologist told them Peter had minimal brain dysfunction; he is not retarded.

Now Arlene Spiller and her friend Bebe Antell, who also has a brain-injured son, now thirty-two, publish a newsletter, *Perceptions*, for distribution to other parents of children who have learning disabilities. It is published monthly, eight times a year, at a subscription price of $15. For subscription and editorial information, the address is Perceptions, Inc., P. O. Box 142, Millburn, New Jersey 07041.[2]

The fact is that parents learn more from each other and from newsletters than they do from doctors. Sol Gordon, a clinical psychologist, child therapist and director of the Institute for Family Research and Education at Syracuse University, said: "I think the assumption that the professionals know best is not a good

---

[2]Nan Robertson. "A newsletter for parents of the learning-disabled." *The New York Times*. March 6, 1979, p. 46.

assumption. My advice is often sought, but I like the idea of parents supporting and sharing and helping each other ... Social behavior, how to get along in this world, is more important for these children than anything else."[3]

"There isn't a learning disabled child in the world who wouldn't give a right arm for help," declared Dr. Akselsen. "Sometimes they say they don't want help, but that's when everything else has failed for them. After a while when he or she sees that improvement is taking place, the child becomes more anxious to work at correction than are the parents."

The symptoms of brain dysfunctional problems show up in the eyes of the child. The eyes may have parallel vision, so that they will not converge to the cross-eyed position. There could be strabismus, or "lazy eye," where one eye turns out. The youngster will usually suffer from eye strain that is noticeable by the parent. More subtle, but frequently seen in learning disabilities, is the inability of the child's eyes to follow a moving target without jerky eye motions.

To test the child, ask him or her to focus on the top of a pencil which is held about two feet from the nose, and move it horizontally back and forth to the extreme of the youngster's direct vision, without allowing the head to move. Then move the pencil upward as high as the child can see it. Next, drop it down to the lowest point to which he can still see the pencil without moving his head. Keep a close watch on the eyes. Notice if they jerk or jump as the child attempts to follow the pencil even when you are moving it quite slowly. If they do, this and other symptoms are possible signs of minimal brain dysfunction.

We'll have a great deal more to say about vision and eyesight in the next chapter.

Chronic depression is another sign. In the April 1979 issue of the *American Journal of Psychiatry*, Irving

---

[3]*Ibid.*

Philips, M.D., director of child and adolescent psychiatry at the University of California Medical Center in San Francisco, reported that depressed infants may be withdrawn and apathetic and fail to thrive. Pre-schoolers may have trouble separating from their parents, appear hyperactive, and show learning disabilities. In the elementary grades, depressed children commonly complain about a host of physical and emotional hurts. They tend to be self-deprecating and overly sensitive and have trouble forming relationships with their peers. They may become the class clowns or daydream in school, fail to recognize their scholastic potential or refuse to go to school altogether.

Adolescents may show more classic signs of depression such as loss of appetite or sudden overeating, sleep disturbances, neglect of school work and personal appearance, extreme uncommunicativeness and avoidance of social interactions. Or their depression, too, may be masked as, for example, extreme hostility and aggressiveness, serious risk-taking or promiscuous sexual behavior. Some have hallucinations or obsessions about death, guilt, hopelessness, failure, humiliation, or worthlessness.

There is a five-part examination to evaluate a child with a learning disability. Dennis P. Cantwell, M.D., Associate Professor of Psychiatry at the University of California, Los Angeles (UCLA) School of Medicine, said you must first get a clear picture of the actual disorder, which he described as an "attention deficit disorder." Second, you should determine if there are special difficulties in learning to read, in language, or in arithmetic. Third, are there specific physical problems, such as asthma, epilepsy, or actual evidence of brain damage? Fourth, is there a family history of similar difficulties? Fifth, what is the child's intelligence? Is a low intelligence quotient compounding the problem?

Objective tests developed by Canadian researchers Marcel Kinsbourne, M.D., Ph.D. and James Swanson,

M.D. help determine the extent of a child's learning and behavior problems.

"Relatively simple but carefully controlled testing procedures minimize therapeutic errors in diagnosing and treating children referred for professional help with specific learning and behavior problems," Dr. Kinsbourne told medical journalists and physicians at another medical symposium we attended in Portland, Oregon on "New Approaches to Minimal Brain Dysfunction, Hyperactivity, and Learning Disabilities," in December 1978. Kinsbourne is Senior Physician, Hospital for Sick Children and Professor of Pediatrics, University of Toronto Faculty of Medicine.

In another instance, Columbia University College of Physicians and Surgeons' professor of clinical psychiatry Richard A. Gardner, M.D. has developed two additional diagnostic tests. The first of his tests measures a child's ability to hold his hand steady over a significant period. The child is asked to place a stylus approximately one-eighth of an inch in diameter inside a hole approximately one-quarter of an inch in diameter for three one-minute periods without touching the sides of the hole.

"Every time the stylus touches the side of the hole, a tone sounds and a clock records the total duration of 'touch time.' Meanwhile, a second clock times each of three trial periods," Dr. Gardner explained. "The test is very sensitive to hyperactivity and impairment in the ability to sustain attention." Accordingly, many MBD children will do poorly."

Dr. Gardner's second examination, a test of letter and number reversal frequency, is given in two parts. "Most children have trouble reading letters that are mirror images and confuse p's and q's, d's and b's, until about age six or seven. This problem usually corrects itself by the time they reach the second grade, but normal children do exhibit some reversals at later ages. Children with MBD, however, usually have this problem for a longer period of time." Dr. Gardner has collected letter reversal frequency data on 500 normal and 350 MBD children.

The first part of the test measures frequency of reversals on execution. The child is asked to write a series of numbers and letters as they are dictated to him. The number of reversals the child makes is compared to normal and MBD children.

In the second part of the test, which measures reversal recognition, the child is presented with a page of letters and numbers. The child is instructed to write an "X" over the incorrect letters and numbers. Dr. Gardner said that the results are then compared with what has been established as "normal" for children of various ages and sex.

Realizing that the child is suffering from a learning disability or MBD, procedures for correction may then be instituted.

Procedures for Correcting Learning Disabilities

"Some have said that the single most common disorder seen by child psychiatrists, psychologists and neurologists is the 'attentional deficit syndrome with learning disorders' or 'minimal cerebral dysfunction,' as it is also called," said Michael E. Cohen, M.D., Associate Professor of Neurology and Pediatricts at the State University of New York at Buffalo School of Medicine.

"Typically, youngsters with this syndrome are boys who are believed to have a dysfunction in motor activity, coordination, attention, cognitive function, impulse control, interpersonal relationships, and responsiveness to social influences," Dr. Cohen clarified. He agreed that the symptoms may arise from genetic variations, biochemical irregularities, perinatal brain insults or other illnesses or injuries sustained during the years which are critical for the development and maturation of the central nervous system, or from unknown causes.

He also observed that the various specialists who see

the child focus on the syndrome from the particular point of view of their own specialty, so that the orthodox child psychiatrist may see it as indicative of a seriously disturbed child, the orthomolecular psychiatrist may see it as a nutritional deficiency, and the allergist may suspect that an environmental toxin or food additive is the basis for the problem. The pharmacologist, neurophysiologist, and to some extent the neurologist, Dr. Cohen added, view this as "an organic syndrome resulting from abnormal balance or neurotransmitter function."

The result is that there have been many different approaches developed for treatment of the child who is learning disabled. The treatment varies with the specialty training of the individual doctor the parents consult, and if one medical discipline fails to confront the problem adequately another is tried. This is what causes parents to shunt their learning disabled children from doctor to doctor, spending thousands of dollars in the process.

Not only do the children get experimented on —treatment by trial and error — but many physicians in the business of treating the mind and emotions don't want anything to do with hyperactive and learning disabled patients. For example, R. Glen Green, M.D., an orthomolecular physician in general practice for thirty-one years in Prince Albert, Saskatchewan, Canada, said at the Second Annual Conference of the Canadian Association for Children with Learning Disabilities: "When I went to medical school, hyperactivity was a rare disease. Certainly teachers feel and know there is an increase; the real question is why. We do not recognize or accept anything, unless it is within the realm of our own experience. Many doctors do not want to be involved with these children. They pass off the child and the parents by saying, 'Oh, he's just a real boy, he'll grow out of it.'"[4]

---

[4]R. Glen Green. "Hyperactivity and the learning disabled child." *J. Orthomolecular Psychiatry* 9:93-104, Second Quarter 1980.

Therefore, while many procedures to correct learning disabilities exist, in this book we will discuss the one method that involves itself wtih coordination correction through exercise — especially the method of *reboundology.

Alfhild Akselsen, Ph.D. has developed a series of tests and movement activities to aid youngsters with coordination problems and learning disabilities. The tests show a child's lack of rhythm, his problem with timing, strength or agility, or the more serious difficulties associated with brain damage. Dr. Akselsen's investigation in the learning disabled field has allowed her to slowly and painstakingly develop some muscle control movements to overcome those various coordination problems. They definitely include the application of rebounding aerobics, with special emphasis on the use of a rebound device having a double suspension system. Rebounding supplies corrective exercises for slow learners and retarded children, alike.

"Rebounding should start in nursery school," said Dr. Akselsen. "I see mind/body improvement occur throughout the growth period of the human organism. When I work with a child who has all kinds of coordination problems culminating in learning disabilities it means he or she has not worked with the gross and fine motor nerve/muscle coordinates. A child should do this from at least first or second grade. I have put rebounding devices in schools not only around the United States but also in schools around the world. The children have to be given a chance to learn up to their capacities. I don't say they'll all end up being geniuses, but they will coordinate their senses up to their own inborn intelligence."

Dr. Akselsen was a school psychologist in Norway more than forty years ago. She had responsibility for learning disabled children for whom everything available was done to bring them into normality. In some

*See page iii

cases, she met failure. With one little boy who was absolutely unable to do what he was supposed to, something pushed the psychologist into requesting the child to walk backwards. He walked three steps and fell on the floor. For the first time, she realized that this type of child does not know left from right or front from back. Such children only recognize a forward direction. From this point onward, Dr. Akselsen knew that coordination, balance and rhythm through exercising, was called for. She has worked with exercises ever since.

"I came upon the use of rebounding equipment by experimenting with many different devices made of wood. For a long time I employed something called the 'trampoline board,' a twelve-foot-long plank, twelve inches wide and two inches thick, that had to be placed eight inches from the floor. It was made of a special springy wood. The children jumped on this plank to get the spring. Other plywood forms also gave spring. Then I began to use ordinary trampolines.

"One day, while I was visiting with Victor Green at his Tri-Flex manufacturing plant and asked that a special type of rebound unit be made. I found he already had it available. This baby form of trampoline works best," Dr. Akselsen said.

Now she is working with mentally retarded infants with IQ's as low as twenty-five. Using massage, exercises, and rebounding, she is succeeding with these babies.

Why does the rebounding device work for improving the body/mind connection? "Because when you are rebounding, you are moving and exercising every brain cell as you are each of the other body cells. Toxic heavy metals are leached out of these brains cells to free up the neurons to work more effectively. Better nourishment has a chance to penetrate the cell walls, too. Furthermore, rebounding has you work from the outside, from the nerve endings toward the brain," said Dr. Akselsen. "That's what I think it does. We don't know for certain, of course, but I can't see the results any other way. I am trying to build a sense of the truth, at this time."

In general, Dr. Akselsen is working with children who are ignored by society — sometimes hidden away in institutions — and turns them into whatever are their mental capacities. In many cases, these learning disabled people turn out to be above average and exceptional human beings. Their primary problem is actually a neuromuscular dysfunction — not reduced intelligence — that prevents them from releasing the information stored within. Dr. Akselsen merely trains the body to respond to the brain. The training involves the eyes, nose, larynx, tongue, fingers, and other organs so that learning disabled persons can finally get to read, write, see properly, speak, and manipulate their muscles in order to put to use the information they have been gathering in all of their lives.

Witnesses tell of seeing children previously unable to speak during fifteen or sixteen years of life — using only three or four words accompanied by grunts to express themselves — in a month or two opening up with full sentences, complete paragraphs, and competent expressions of thoughts, following a program of coordinated exercises, *reboundology, massage, neuro-muscular training, and testing done by Alfhild Akselsen, Ph.D.

Her entire technique is concerned with teaching the body to respond to the brain's output. When the physical defect is corrected, the mental defect is also corrected. There are multiple places in the body where there may be a neurological short circuit. When it affects a muscle, the brain's command to the left hand to move may cause the right hand to move. Or, the left hand may move but also the left foot comes along with it. Or, the child's eye may twitch, or nothing may happen.

The learning disabled person lives in his or her own small, private Hell!

The person knows what's happening to him. He

---

*See pg. iii

knows that others are making a judgment of his actions so as to believe eventually that the person doesn't know anything.

Dr. Akselsen's work is helping these learning disabled people to free themselves from their physical handicaps, which most of the time are diagnosed as mentally retarded, brain damaged, or antisocially behaving. They may show no brain damage on an electroencephalogram (EEG) or no lumpy brain area on the computerized axial tomograph (CAT) scan, thus offering no clinical evidence of brain damage.

A chapter in a book such as this cannot do justice to the Akselsen techniques, but we shall endeavor to enlighten you a little on some of her procedures. She uses rebound exercise units, giant trampolines, deep nerve massage, light sensory massage, excellent nutrition, and a lot more. Rebound International, Inc. of South Houston, Texas, using the Tri-Flex Manufacturing Company facilities, is a layperson group of volunteers actively engaged in carrying on Dr. Akselsen's work.

The following are some of the testing procedures applied:

A. With the child lying on his back, legs extended, feet together, arms at sides, you analyze his ability to stay in a place in a straight line. Correct any deviation from a straight position.

B. In the same position as A above, the child lifts his head and turns it to the right and left.

C. The child stands, bent forward at the waist, hands on knees, legs straight, and rotates the head right and left.

D. Lying on his back, the child raises one arm and while watching it, rotates this arm in a circular motion in one direction and then another; repeating with the other arm.

E. The child bounces on the rebound unit while his eyes are affixed on one spot.

F. Lying on his back, the child watches an object

suspended by a string from the ceiling as it swings in a circle.

G. Lying on his back, the child raises one leg with the knee stiff and watches his foot while he rotates his leg in one direction and then the other; alternating legs.

H. While on his back, the child rolls in a straight line.

I. Lying flat on the stomach with head raised, the child crawls forward using hands, feet, elbows and knees for movement.

J. The child rises to his hands and knees and crawls forward across the floor. Then he crawls backward.

K. Lying flat on the back, the child lifts one leg slowly with the knee stiff; repeating with the other leg. Then he lifts both legs slowly together.

L. The child performs sit-ups with legs extended and feet together, first with the fingers touching the toes and then with the hands folded behind the head.

M. The child performs push-ups.

N. The child performs a push-up with the hands turned inward, fingertips touching.

O. The child does sit-ups and stand-ups while holding the arms crossed over the chest.

P. The child walks in a coordinated manner.

Q. The child stands with his back against a wall, eyes affixed to a spot on the opposite wall, arms held straight out, and walks across the room by touching the heel to the toe of each foot with each step. Then he backs up the same way.

R. The above testing procedure is repeated with the arms out to the side, the hands on the head, or the eyes closed.

S. The child does all of the above walking on a balance beam, two inches by four inches wide, with the eyes open.

T. With feet together and arms slightly bent at the elbows, the child stands and hops on a carpeted floor or on a rebounding device. In a series of short jumps, he hops forward and backward.

U. The child repeats the hops on the rebound unit but

on just one foot and then on the other.

V. The child jumps straight up and down three times, either on the floor or on the rebound device.

W. The child performs jumping jacks either on the floor or on the rebound device.

X. The child balances on one leg for one minute, first with eyes open and then with eyes closed.

Confirmation of Learning Disability Improvement from Rebounding

A statement written by Mrs. Florence M. Franet, teacher of aphasic students, Mount Diablo Unified School District, Concord, California, says the following:

> ... I purchased a rebound unit for my own use and that of my family. I felt so well as a result of using it, I wanted to share it with my students, too. Transporting it back and forth from home to school everyday became a real chore, so I purchased a second one for the specific use of students in the school's handicap program. This rebound unit was used as a source for daily activities and exercise in my classroom for special education of aphasic students during the 1976-77 school year. Six students ages eight and nine participated starting in September 1976.
>
> The students began using the rebound unit by just trying to stand and balancing themselves on it. Then they bounced with two feet together and then jogging easily. Three of the students were able to bounce by themselves from the start, but the other three had to be assisted. Gradually all could bounce alone and begin the exercises, although the most severely involved student took nine days before she could even stand alone. Let us take time to follow this student's development.
>
> At the beginning of this school year Frances could not coordinate her small motor development enough to draw a circle or copy a single letter. She did attempt to write her first name, but one had to know what Frances was attempting in order to read it (///-c'/). Her eye/hand coordination was nill. Her speech was unintelligible. She used only small words and sometimes short phrases.
>
> After one month of using the rebound unit, Frances

was bouncing with two feet by herself. Following this, she developed sufficient coordination to run slowly on the rebound unit. In four months, Fran was running and dancing on it. Her language developed along with this. In four month's time you could also read her name when she wrote it. She could draw circles. In six months, she could trace the letters of her last name. In eight months she could copy her last name. In nine months she could write it by herself. She was able to write some other letters, too, by this time. Needless to say, she was a very happy little girl and Fran's parents were pleased, as well.

Frances's verbal expression developed along with her written and motor expression. She was using simple sentences, gradually extending them into whole paragraphs by the end of these nine months. Her receptive language improved also.

Another student whose large motor development was fairly well coordinated, could bounce and jog on the rebounder but could not hop on either foot alone without losing his balance. George's verbal expressive language consisted of phrases and sentences without verbs. His comprehension receptive language was impaired.

After George used the rebound unit for five months, he could hop on either foot for 300 to 400 counts. After six months he could jump rope on the device. After another month he was skipping rope on it. His expressive verbal language developed considerably during this time. His receptive language improved by about two-and-a-half to three years.

All of these students showed growth in their coordination, language skills, health, and attitudes. I had expected to see growth for these students and had worked with aphasic students for five years previously to working with this group. but this growth far exceeded expectations. I attribute their additional gains and development and total stimulation to the use of the rebound unit.

In the 1977-78 school year, I used the rebound unit with high school-age aphasic students. Again, I saw beautiful development in physical coordination, muscle development, self-concept, and language skills. We fitted the use of the rebound unit into the mathematics and social studies program. A four-inch cross is painted on the classroom wall representing north, east, south, and west directions. It's placed at eye level. The assignment often was to bounce 360 times divided equally while facing each of the four directions.

Some of the better coordinated aphasic boys decided to challenge one another to see who could hop on one foot standing on the rebound unit the most number of times. They started out with 100, then 300, then 700, then 1000. It was getting too difficult for them to count the number of hops accurately. Therefore, they used a stopwatch and set a five-minute period for themselves. Each of three boys could hop on one foot but not the other. So each would challenge himself to develop his weaker side. One boy did it in three weeks; the second did it in seven weeks; the third finally mastered the alternate side after more than six months.

I would like to see all handicapped students have the opportunity to have use of a rebound unit on a daily basis. It would minimize their handicaps more rapidly.

9

Rebounding Aerobics to Revitalize Vision

From the age of two, the author of this book, Dr. Morton Walker, has had to wear eyeglasses for structural vision assistance.

My original problem was an imbalance of one or more of the six muscles controlling the movements of each eye so that my left eye was pulled out of alignment. Crossed eyes (esotropia) resulted. From my mother, additionally, I inherited abnormally short eyeballs, resulting in a tendency to farsightedness (hyperopia). The uncrossed right eye gradually was taking over the major load of seeing until my left eye finally was corrected with lenses. The right has remained dominant. The farsightedness was also assisted in my early years by corrective lenses, and I remember growing up repeatedly having eyeglasses replaced because they were frequently broken in play.

Complicating my seeing clearly, later as an adult, was my development of a third defect. It also belonged to this group of eye troubles arising from variations in the shape of the eyeball. Astigmatism is a vision condition in which images at all distances may be distorted or blurred. Astigmatism is not a disease and no particular time of life is characteristic of when it's most likely to occur. For me, the problem arose in my mid-thirties when the shape of the front of the eye became more oval than round. Exactly why this happens is not known, but some theories say it is an inherited condition or caused as the eye develops. Other theories blame such factors as poor lighting, incorrect posture or increased amounts of close work. The latter may have been my case, because I had previously practiced as a foot surgeon performing my operations with tiny incisions on the toes. My astigmatism was also corrected by prescription lenses.

At age forty, another natural defect, presbyopia, the inability to focus the eyes clearly on close objects, came upon me. Presbyopia is known as an inevitable result of aging. I eventually had to change my lenses and wear bifocals.

From age forty to fifty, there was no alteration in my ability to see except that each lens diopter, the unit used to measure the light-bending power of a lense, steadily was increased for both of my eyes. My lenses were growing thicker and stronger as my eyes grew weaker and more accommodative to the structural corrections.

Suddenly, in February 1980, I found myself unable to see well out of my right eye, the one I had always depended upon to tell what was reality in the world around me. In fact, even while wearing eyeglasses, I had to close the right eye to see what was on a movie screen or to see down the road while driving for reading traffic signs ahead. I was puzzled by discovering I could see at a distance better with my right eye by removing my eyeglasses. It was then I realized I needed a new lens, weaker or stronger, depending upon the optometrist's examination.

It turned out that I required a full diopter reduction in the correction for farsightedness, and my presbyopia and astigmatism corrections had to be lessened, as well. A new elasticity in the crystalline lens of my dominant right eyeball was being restored. There was no change needed in the left eye correction. The traditional structural optometrist who examined me had absolutely no explanation as to why my one eye should suddenly revert to more youthful functioning.

In searching my lifestyle there was just one alteration I could distinguish as a change from the usual way I lived. For the prior year, I had been vigorously engaging in rebounding aerobics — not for its effect on vision — but to enhance my daily cardiovascular exercise program. During this period, I had been writing *How Not to Have a Heart Attack* (Franklin Watts, Inc., 1980) and had included in the book a description of the training effect derived from rebound exercise. Rebounding worked well to help reverse hardening of the arteries. Since I do what I write about and write about what I do, I performed rebounding aerobics. Never did I dream it would improve my eyesight, but it did and is continuing the improvement.

We will have more to say about why this improvement takes place later in this chapter.

The Real Reason We Wear Eyeglasses

According to the National Health Survey,[1] some 94 million Americans wear some kind of corrective lenses. These are civilians, three years of age and older, not living in institutions.

About 2.1 percent wear contact lenses, mainly young adults between the ages of seventeen and twenty-four.

Corrective lenses are worn by more women than men, by more office workers than laborers, and the proportion of the population wearing glasses increases with age and income.

More than 3 million Americans suffer vision-stealing cataracts. Color blindness, a hereditary condition

[1]*Characteristics of Persons with Corrective Lenses*, U.S., 1971. Series 10, No. 93. DHEW Publication No. 75-1520. Washington: USGPO, 1974.

which cannot be altered by treatment, affects almost 2 million; 797,000 have glaucoma; and, 145,000 suffer detachment of the retina. In addition, almost 10 million U.S. citizens say they have trouble seeing.[2]

Among the nation's 24 million children, six to eleven years of age: 10 percent have a disease condition or other abnormality in one or both eyes; 10 percent wear glasses; 9 percent have infections; and 8 percent blink or frequently rub them while reading.[3]

Of the country's nearly 23 million youths ages twelve to seventeen years, 8 million wear glasses and another 10 million need glasses. A fifth of those who wear eyeglasses need to have them changed.

Nearly 2 million youths have significant eye abnormalities, the major condition being strabismus (also known as "wall eye," "wandering eye," and "cross eye"), which afflicts 800,000.[4][5]

Have you ever wondered why so many people need to wear eyeglasses or contact lenses? Does this mean we are really a nation made up largely of people with impaired vision? Is the human eye not the best of all possible eyes in the Animal Kingdom?

While the human eye does not see as far as the eagle's nor see as well in the dark as the owl's, nor as well in water as a fish's, it is one of the most versatile eyes nature has ever made. It sees stereoscopic, 3-D color moving pictures from one side of you to the other. It adapts to a very wide range of darkness and brightness, and it can keep objects in focus, though they change distance.

Really, only one true reason exists for so many of us to wear eyeglasses.

---

[2]*Prevalence of Selected Impairments, U.S.*, 1971, Series 10, No. 99. DHEW Publication No. (HRA) 75-1526. Washington: USGPO, 1975.

[3]*Eye Examination Findings Among Children, U.S.* Series 11, No. 115. DHEW Publication No. (HSM) 72-1057. Washington: USGPO, 1972.

[4]*Eye Examination Findings Among Youths Aged 12-17 Years, U.S.* Series 11, No. 155. DHEW Publication No. (HRA) 76-1627. Washington: USGPO, 1975.

[5]*Refraction Status of Youths 12-17 Years, U.S.*, Series 11, No. 148. DHEW Publication No. (HRA) 75-1630. Washington: USGPO, 1974.

At a particular time in your life it's possible that a professional authority, an ophthalmologist, or optometrist, will tell you to wear eyeglasses. An opthalmologist, also called an oculist, is a medical doctor trained in the diagnosis and treatment of eye diseases and correction of optical errors. An optometrist is trained to test the eyes for nonmedical defects of vision in order to prescribe and dispense corrective lenses. Ophthalmologists and optometrists don't often involve themselves in exercise and nutrition when they prescribe for their patients. Their primary skill is to be able to determine how your eyes are functioning immediately at the moment of being tested. They seldom predict what your eyes are going to be like in the future.

Upon having your eyes tested, you may hear the statement that you must have specific lenses at this time to correct your vision to where you can see as well as possible with the eye problem you possess. Yet, in a short time, if you remove some stress from your life or take better nutrition or exercise your body or experience other positive and healthful occurrences in your lifestyle, your vision could markedly improve spontaneously.

A lot of people, for instance, wear eyeglasses because they are under prolonged stress of a mental, emotional, physical, chemical, or thermal nature. They feel better by getting lens assistance for their eyes. They use less energy this way. Others wear eyeglasses because their occupations have them staring at the printed page all day. Still more people, because of a vitamin deficiency, a smoking habit, an addiction to alcohol, or some other destructive condition must wear eyeglasses. Some women find themselves feeling better during menstruation from the support given by their lenses.

If you happen to have an eye examination during a time that your body is in a state of disrepair, the resulting response by the eyes will be captured in glass lenses. The eyes are so related to different parts of the body that if anything goes wrong with any body part, the eyes will be among the first organs to show weakness or ill health. Not knowing she is pregnant, if a women who has newly conceived visits an optometrist or ophthalmologist for an eye examination, he or she will be able to tell the woman of her pregnancy through looking into her eyes with ocular instruments.

Thus, some people who have been ill, realizing it or not, are wearing glasses because their eyes were checked during their period of acute body weakness. Over time, they will have adjusted to their lenses and such wearing becomes part of their lifestyle. They will not have solved a health problem but merely covered over one set of its symptoms.

Many times, the prescribing of eyeglasses is empirical treatment for symptomatic disease. Seldom do eyeglasses permanently solve a problem with vision.

Moreover, the link between poor vision and poor nutrition has been proven by Ben Lane, O.D. of Lake Hiawatha, New Jersey. Dr. Lane is chairman of the Nutrition Committee, College of Optometrists in Vision Development and has long been connecting how people see to what they eat.

At the May 1980 conference of the American College of Advancement in Medicine held in Reno, Nevada, Dr. Lane told us there are numerous instances in which it is known that poor diet caused myopia (nearsightedness). For example, a pregnant woman who drinks alcoholic beverages of more than two ounces a day will produce a child with congenital myopia.

And the impact of diet on myopia is even more subtle than intoxication in pregnancy. "The problems begin," Dr. Lane said in a prior newspaper interview, "when people are required to handle close work for prolonged periods of time — day after day — for more than a two-week period. This can start in childhood, when kids have learned to read and now read to learn. The eye accommodates to this stress by an elevation of intraocular pressure, which in turn enlarges the eyeball. This makes it easier to focus at close distances without the eye having to work so hard.

"Normally, the enlargement causes no real problems. A small amount of nearsightedness results, but only as much as is useful. But when nearsightedness is combined with poor nutrition," Dr. Lane warned, "this adjustive mechanism of the eyes produces an exaggerated effect. When a number of nutrients are missing or deficient, the body has trouble in controlling intraocular pressure. The relevant nutrients are the vitamins that are easily destroyed by heat, such as vitamins C, B-2, B-6, B-15, pantothenic acid, and choline. All are water soluble and are often lost in processing.

"Then, when other nutrients are lacking, the eye responds to short periods of intraocular pressure by distending too easily. And this results," Dr. Lane said, "in too large an increase in myopia. The relevant nutrients in this instance are calcium, vitamin D, and other supporting factors such as vitamin A and zinc."

What is the result? The myopia is recognized finally by a parent or teacher, and the child is taken to the eye doctor to have his vision checked. The question of nutrition hardly ever comes up as part of the case history in an optometric or ophthalmologic examination. Invariably, corrective lenses are prescribed, instead. The nutritionally deficient child is destined to wear eyeglasses the rest of his life to correct nearsightedness when all the time some fresh vegetables, fruit, dairy products, and a few vitamins would have done the job permanently.

To test the bonds between nutrition and myopia, Dr. Lane took the case histories of 100 of his own patients. In each instance, he did a complete nutritional workup. He also asked each patient to provide him with a hair sample, which he had analyzed for mineral content. He found that those who were nearsighted had about one-third the amount of chromium in their hair. He also discovered that myopic youngsters between the ages of seven and seventeen had a lot of calcium in their hair, compared to children with normal vision.

The analysis of diet showed that the nearsighted

tended to consume a far higher ration of refined carbohydrates such as sugar and white bread to other carbohydrates. The nearsighted's ratio was 35.27 percent,
compared to 9.61 percent for the farsighted. He also
found that the nearsighted person whose visual problem was growing was eating large amounts of denatured
or overcooked protein, three times the recommended
daily allowance.

How does this nutrition and vision fit together? Biochemistry is involved.

Dr. Lane explained that an intake of sugar depletes
the body's reserve of chromium, so the decrease in
chromium would indicate an effect of the sugar. Also,
sugar acts as an "anti-vitamin," destroying the nutrients that help control intraocular pressure.

Furthermore, eating protein that has been cooked
beyond 130 to 140 degrees fahrenheit makes vitamin
B-6 unavailable for body use. This also results in the
loss of pantothenic acid. "Devitaminization such as this
means poorer control of eye pressure," said Dr. Lane.
"The high calcium levels in the hair would be the result of too much cooked protein. Denatured proteins
wash calcium out of the body into the urine and into
the hair. Lower levels are absorbed by other body tissues, including the eye. And calcium is one of the nutrients required to control distension in the eye."[6]

Dr. Lane said that his studies point to the need for a
diet rich in foods that have not lost their original vitamins and trace mineral constituents. We all have the requirement for more raw fruits and vegetables and for
less fish and meat — unless they are served extremely
rare. Try improving your nutrition before you accept the
wearing of eyeglasses for the correction of nearsightedness, or other such problems.

---

[6]Peggy Carroll. "Poor nutrition, vision linked." *Sunday Daily Record,* September
2, 1979, p. 22.

Visual Therapists Differ from Structural Optometrists

From the description of how Ben Lane, O.D. practices as compared to an ordinary optometrist who just prescribes lenses for the empirical treatment of eye symptoms, it becomes obvious that two therapeutic philosophies are in conflict here. In fact, there are conventional, structural optometrists and new school, developmental optometrists. Structural optometrists consider vision as a circumstance of living without any connection to the total well being of a person. Developmental optometrists tie vision to a person's life experience that engages both the brain and the nervous system. Whereas conventional optometrists correct vision with lenses and believe the correction continues only while you wear those lenses, the developmental optometrist uses visual training and other holistic approaches (along with lenses) to develop in the person a higher level of visual efficiency.

Of about 25,000 practicing optometrists in the United States, only approximately 800 use methods of visual therapy. These methods are less lucrative and more time consuming for the doctor than the prescribing and selling of eyeglasses.

Albert Shankman, O.D. of Norwalk, Connecticut, is a developmental optometrist who specializes in vision training that includes body awareness, postural correction, and an attempt to have patients induce changes in processing what and how they see. We interviewed Dr. Shankman in his home in the summer of 1980. From him we learned that vision is part of the mental processing of the individual. In order to have consistency between what is seen and the way a person believes it should be, the individual changes his visual functioning to develop any combination of visual and eye conditions, such as nearsightedness, astigmatism, farsightedness, ignoring one of the images of double vision, and other eye compensations. These usually develop in combination with a postural and/or biophysical change.

The vision therapist does a vision analysis to measure the adaptations and anomalies which have been built in by constant repetition of the individual attempting to change the way objects look into the way he thinks they "should look," in order to be consistent with his adaptations. A structural optometrist does this analysis also, but he makes his corrections solely with lenses. The vision therapist uses lenses, improved nutrition, and eye exercises, including the rebounder.

Dr. Shankman said, "Vision training practiced as a full spectrum optometric technique attempts to change the way one interprets inputs from all the senses for a better match with real time and space. Sometimes, as inputs are processed more realistically, there are dramatic alterations in individual behavior that take place internally and can trigger other unintentional changes. Often, they are very drastic for a person and can be traumatic. All changes have a definite impact on the person's lifestyle, and are usually observed by someone else before the individual is aware of them. But, most of the time personal alterations in behavior are usually for the better and unintentional. In other words, it is not a change toward making life more acceptable to the person because he is told that a certain prescribed behavior is the way to make life more acceptable. His behavior change is made as a byproduct of an altered perspective of life. The individual adjusts his personality to become more consistent with the new perspective."

Thus, vision training can bring on a new way of looking at the world and a new way of life. In vision training, the patient makes his behavior changes without realizing that he is making them, and they are usually in the direction of seeing more realistically. Vision training develops a better perceived relationship between the body and mind. When a poor relationship exists, Dr. Shankman describes his patient as suffering from "dysrelatia". His term stems from the Greek prefix *dys* (difficult) and the Latin word *relatia* (relationships), meaning "difficulty in forming relationships."

Visual therapists differ from structural optometrists by assisting the patient to self-initiate relationships to the surroundings efficiently and automatically. The structural optometrist on the other hand, is nothing more than an educated mechanic who sets in place the best lens to allow the patient's eyes to adjust to the light images they take in. He gives no consideration to dysrelatia but merely treats the human eye as a light-proof globe with a window at the front. In this globe, light is gathered by a living crystal dome, the **cornea,** which arches over a space containing a watery liquid called the **aqueous** circulating below it.

That "the eye is the mirror of the soul" is more than a poetic statement; for its functions are affected by emotional and physical health. The blood vessels inside the eye are the only ones which can be directly seen in the body without any surgery. This enables the eye doctor to discover clues to bodily conditions such as high blood pressure, hardening of the arteries, and diabetes. The eye also yields clues to general systemic diseases such as liver disease, infections, brain tumors, skin diseases, and nutritional deficiencies.

The visual therapist uses a variety of neuromuscular exercises similar to the ones applied in the coordination correction of learning disabled children that we described in chapter eight. The rebound unit is one of the therapeutic tools sometimes used by the vision therapist to help the eyes carry accurate information through the optic nerve and to the brain.

How the Eyes Carry on Their Function

Before describing how rebounding exercise works advantageously to bring about vision therapy and more perfect eyesight, we should first briefly explain the functioning of the eye and how it carries information to the brain for interpretation.

The cornea concentrates light from the world outside into the crystalline lens that covers the opening of the dark chamber of the eye. The purpose of the lens is to focus light rays so as to cast a sharp image on the retina at the back of the interior of the eye. A ring of circular and radiating muscle fibers manipulate the lens, changing its shape. The lens is pulled flat to bring close objects into focus.

Images fall on the paper-thin retina, which lines the back two-thirds of the eye's inner surface. The light image stimulates the retina's 127 million rods and cones, which send tiny electrical signals to the brain, where images are received and interpreted.

Electrochemical mechanisms in the retina allow it to adapt to over 100,000-fold brightness-to-darkness light intensities. Some of this is due to the detection of bright light by the cones and of dim light by the rods. Also, each of these microscopic structures has internal adjustments, as well.

In front of the lens is the magic ring of muscle by which we tell a person's eye color, the iris. This iris is a diaphragm with a hole in the center, the pupil. The pupil narrows and widens continuously and automatically, to let more light into the eye, or hold back light.

Only two and a half centimeters wide, the human eye is a miracle of miniaturization which accomplishes far more than any television camera many times its size. Complex networks of blood vessels and nerves serve its electrochemical needs. In addition, it sends its image through the optic nerve to the brain, where the sense of sight actually occurs. The mind takes over.

Dr. Shankman points out that the mind has four functions with no function independent of the other or acting in isolation from the others. "The first function of the mind is as a collector of impressions as well as a recollector of impressions," he wrote in a continuing education course created for the Optometric Extension

Program.[7] "The second function of the mind is that of determination. This determination results in the mental experience of knowing, feeling, willing, and motivating, which helps to develop knowledge. The third function of the mind is the one that helps an individual to experience and then stores that experience as knowledge which is useful or meaningful. The fourth function of the mind is what takes place as perception. The four functions must take place so that problems are solved and decisions made. This is the process of how the mind thinks.

"The speed of the thinking process depends on how quickly the steps are made from stimulus to perception," wrote Dr. Shankman. "The mind is activated through the sensory organs. The manner in which the sensory inputs are used depends on the individual's past experience in making mental relationships of sensory inputs.

"The mind is also stimulated by what some call senses of action. These actions are grasping, speaking, walking, excretion, and sexual activity. The mind becomes more sensitive to the sensory stimuli as one develops greater body awareness. Greater body awareness develops more efficient thinking skills. It is a synergistic action, so if one improves, the other will improve automatically. That is why any program that uses the body properly, helps one develop better thinking skills, which then transfers to their total lifestyle. Using the body properly, then, becomes the commonality in all the therapy programs."

Dr. Shankman is part of a group of developmental optometrists, specialists within the optometric profession, who perform visual therapy. Some of them make effective use of rebounding aerobics for the improvement of vision. Body awareness is the key to their success, in many instances.

---

[7] Albert Shankman. "Dysrelatia." *Vision Training*. Continuing Education Courses, Vol. 52 (Duncan, Oklahoma: Optometric Extension Program, 1980), pp. 31 & 32.

Rebounding Aerobics for Vision Therapy

Theodore S. Kadet, O.D., a vision therapist in Issaquah, Washington, has found the techniques of rebounding aerobics to be valuable for using the eye muscles to correct contractions of the cornea. Dr. Kadet said, "Rebounding creates an awareness of using vision as a primary guiding system for movement. The inability to use vision efficiently as a major sentry system to the brain can be a primary cause of learning disabilities in children and adults. I am confirming what other authorities have found before me. Our treatment in optometry of these visual perception dysfunctions help Mother Nature along in the development of vision and vision-auditory interaction systems."

Vision therapists, spearheaded by notables in the field such as A.M. Skeffington, O.D., G.N. Getman, O.D., and D.B. Harmon, Ph.D., under the auspices of the Optometric Extension Program, provide clues to visual difficulties and their correction. Rebound exercise is a main therapeutic approach. It supplies an environment where the perceptual system matures at a more rapid rate.

In explaining the visual therapy, Dr. Kadet said "We concentrate on such areas as visually guided body movements; hand-eye coordination; visual size, space, form and direction relationships; visual-auditory integration; figure-ground relationships; visualization and memory skills. The rebounding device is used to bring about efficient visually guided movement of the entire body. Rebounding aerobics gives magnificent feedback as to what the child did, thus bringing about a rapid awareness as using vision to guide movement.

"Using the rebound unit often helps to bring about directional awareness, especially right and left. Confusion in these areas is a result of letter and word reversals. The device has found a welcome home in the offices of developmental optometrists using vision therapy. It is one of the most effective techniques to bring on visually guided movement pattern," concluded Dr. Kadet.

Dr. G.M. Getman also stated, "Clinical and research studies of rebound exercise indicate that the rebound unit can provide experiences that influence a child's academic success. Optometrists are recommending rebound exercise for the improvements of the total visual and body control."

Dr. Shankman, who recently incorporated rebounding aerobics as part of his visual training program, added, "When I work with patients in optometric vision training, I want them to be able to identify a stimulus and to be aware of any change in the stimulus. Using the body to begin vision training is the best way to start the individual being aware of when there is a change, plus the degree of the change in the action stimuli. The goal of body awareness is to have the patient become aware of the stimulus regardless of its strength, when the smallest change takes place in strength, or change in what it represents."

Use of the rebounding device permits total body awareness of where you are in space. It helps you gather clues from your surroundings so that a habit pattern builds. The habit of knowing where you are in space from clues provides depth perception. You see better and interpret the information coming to your brain through your eyes more effectively.

"In rebounding, you have to learn to use your muscles and do it quickly," said Dr. Shankman. "If you don't learn muscle coordination on the rebounding device, you will face a severe consequence of falling and possibly hurting yourself. Whenever there is a consequence you will learn faster. Rebounding requires that you keep your balance, and you use your eyes for this purpose. By rebounding the same way, using the same exercise positions time after time, you are bound to come to a saturation level where your eyes won't improve anymore. But changing the exercises so as to force yourself into new balancing positions will have the eyes continue their improvement. You get the benefit from rebounding for the sight and mind by relating the objects around you to the space which you are occupying as you bounce up and down. For this purpose, it's better not to watch television while you are rebounding, because you may ignore the rest of the visual field around you."

Dr. Shankman suggested, "Eye improvement might speed up by rebounding to the beat of a metronome. Have the metronome change its rhythm, and you will then get a 'thinking' experience by conforming to the metronome's sound change in your bouncing. You will have feedback from knowing you are rebounding in rhythm correctly."

Raymond Gottlieb, O.D. of Santa Monica, California, another visual therapist, agrees with Dr. Shankman about the rhythm correction of rebounding aerobics. Dr. Gottlieb said, "One of the characteristics of people who suffer from inefficient vision is the lack of rhythm. The rebounding device gives rhythm to the brain from the systematic bouncing. This allows the eyes some externally generated rhythm to fall back on and thus become more coordinated. Your bounce acts like a metronome. You become the metronome yourself.

"Physiologically, you have all of these proprioceptive inputs hitting the thalmus, which is the section of the brain receiving sensory inputs, especially auditory and visual information. Getting multiple inputs, the thalmus organizes the visual readings at a particular moment in time. Also, with the greater circulation stimulated from rebounding, you will have more energy for seeing. There is circulation of the cerebral spinal fluid in the brain, enhanced lymphatic circulation, and better blood circulation. Any toxic circumstances possibly interfering with the vision centers will be dissipated," said Dr. Gottlieb.

"The way the rebound unit is used is a factor, too" he added. "If a therapist acts as an assistant and observer, the rebounding participant will get a lot more benefit out of his bouncing. The therapist helps to monitor progress and himself adds to the feedback from the rebound unit. The observer can show you if your mind wanders by remarking upon an incorrect answer when you produce one while bouncing and reading an eye chart. Rebounding alone, you're not likely to take sufficient responsibility for doing a procedure or eye exercise correctly. Then, you won't learn, or you'll learn poorly," Dr. Gottlieb said.

In working with the rebounding apparatus, a visual therapist helps the patient monitor his own errors and his own perfection. The visual therapist is really attempting to teach a process of seeing and a way of using your brain to assimilate all the information coming into it. It's not mechanical as is done in structural optometry, but rather you are taught a learning style.

Dr. Gottlieb recommended that you try a test to see if you have a coordination or learning problem. If you can bounce on all fours, the two knees and two hands bearing your own weight on the rebound device, and can spring up and down without bucking, you indicate that you have it all together — excellent coordination. Dr. Gottlieb discovered this self-test when he worked at a mental hospital attending to retarded inmates. They could never bounce on all fours.

There are other visual tests and exercises to perform while you're bouncing on the rebound unit. For instance, Dr. Shankman suggests that you could mount the front page of a newspaper on the wall and read smaller and smaller headlines as you rebound. Or, you could read from your own eye chart.

For another exercise, try observing the corner of a room where the ceiling and wall meet and follow where they join all across the room with your eyes as you bounce.

These various suggested techniques are possible ways to strengthen your eyes as you rebound. How? Why? Because the eyes are comprised of body cells, and every cell in the body is basically similar to every other. They come from the same egg and sperm source, have the DNA (deoxyribonucleic acid), know their separate jobs, and read that part of the blueprint of life that has something to do with their job. The cells of the eye know what messages they're supposed to send and receive.

The up-and-down activity of acceleration, deceleration, and gravity develop a greater impact on the eye cells at the bottom of the bounce where every cell is being exercised, stimulated, and doing its job to the best of its ability. Physical cellular strength builds in the millions of eye cells at the bottom of the rebounding bounce.

Furthermore, rebounding permits better aqueous circulation to take place in the eye to feed the cornea, the iris, and the lens. Unlike the rest of the body, the aqueous is a puddle of nutrition for the eye cells. This clear solution has the same chemical makeup as the lymph. It contains nutrients, enzymes, metabolic wastes, and other constituents. An aqueous that circulates more effectively gives you a cleaner and more nourishing environment for the eye cells to do their job.

Rebound exercise eliminates stress, which is a primary reason for people to wear eyeglasses. Like crutches, the lenses reduce the effort for the eye muscles.

When you are stressed, you close down, shrink in, and don't flow with the situation. But Dr. Gottlieb told how he uses the exercises of rebounding to overcome stress. He said, "If you are involved in a stress situation, you follow a characteristic pattern for dealing with that stress. Rebounding exposes the pattern to you and to the therapist, if you're being assisted, and a positive reward is created by the bouncing exercise. You then get to learn your stress pattern very well, thus allowing you to break it and get rid of the stress."

Becoming aware of the movement of your eyes as you bounce, just like a piano player becomes aware of his fingers, tends to give the eyes strength and clarity. You then learn how they can improve. The multiple combination of all these aspects of seeing do provide the basis of better sight and vision.

Regardless of the condition of your eyes, unless they are sightless, they can be improved beyond the vision you currently have. The end result of your applying visual therapy in the form of rebounding aerobics is that better perception comes upon you. Perception is the way in which you look at life and act or react to it. Improved perception has you approach life in a more uplifted way so that you must become a happier person.

In an interview especially for this book, Ann Hoopes, co-author of *Eye Power, The First Report on Visual Training* (Alfred A. Knopf, 1979), told us of her thirty-year-old son, Peter, who became one of those people experiencing improved perception and found himself a happier person.

We'll let Ann Hoopes tell about her child: "My son Peter didn't finish college because he had a terrible time reading and had one injured eye. He finally gave up and turned to carpentry and bartending and other things. His eye disability ran his life because there wasn't anything he could do in the white collar world. He couldn't read easily. Over the past ten years he noticed he was getting progressively unable to read, and he felt dizzy at times and confused. His problem is that he has one eye that sees near and one eye that sees far.

"This is a not-uncommon chronic problem. As a matter of fact, former President Jimmy Carter has this eye problem, which sets up a syndrome in people's thinking when they suffer from this. It makes it difficult for them to make decisions because one eye pulls the brain in a near direction and the other eye pulls in a far direction. This is why I believe President Carter followed so many zigzag foreign policies," said Ann Hoopes.

"Peter, too, has been unable to make decisions about his life. For about five months, now, Peter has been in visual training, and he can finally read comfortably, has taken courses and gotten his real estate license, done some clerical jobs on the side, gone jogging and swimming every day, and is getting his life in order. Peter is filled with a kind of energy that he has never experienced before.

"Twice a week for a year, my son went for visual training to Stanley A. Appelbaum, O.D. of Bethesda, Maryland. He also does some home visual exercises for twenty-five minutes a day and he does a lot of daily physical exercise. Also, he takes good nutrition including many vitamins," Mrs. Hoopes concluded.

In summary, the eyes are semi-muscular organs that must be exercised like any other muscle in the body. The techniques for visual therapy are quite specific eye muscle movements for conditioning the eyes to see more effectively. Oftentimes, the visual therapy includes rebounding aerobics, since rebounding exercises every muscle in the body including the eyes.

10

Techniques of Rebounding Aerobics

Rebounding is an enjoyable and gentle exercise that promotes self-healing of the body and mind. It offers a new style of physical activity that puts more bounce into your life. Rebounding is fun, leads to improved posture, increased vascularity, better muscle tone, enhanced timing, sharper vision, greater coordination, surer balance, more rhythm, elevated energy levels, and holistic living, in general. The movements provide you with freedom to turn, twist, kick, and stretch in the air or on the mat. Such movements are perfectly safe, and they make gravity act as a benefactor. By working against constant gravitational pressure while bouncing, you resist the Earth's pull. Your resistance builds strength. Gravity becomes a force for the good of your entire body.

The main precaution is to start rebounding aerobics gradually. The concentrated exercise activates all the bodily systems simultaneously because of its anti-gravity movements. Your up-and-down motion compresses and decompresses the flesh and fluids of the whole body, all its tissues, organs, and systems, so that wastes will

167

be sucked out of the 60 trillion body cells quickly. Don't let this happen too fast or you'll be unloading more toxins in your bloodstream than you're used to. Excessive beginning rebounding can actually have you feeling lethargic and fatigued from the escape of your own stored cellular toxins. Take it slow and get rid of them gradually.

Our aim is to attain the harmony of health for everyone who brings rebounding into their present and future life. To accomplish such harmony requires a slow and steady workup to the more advanced and therapeutic techniques of this aerobic exercise. Our recommendation is that you adapt the techniques one by one every few days so that three months may pass before all of them are part of your program. DO NOT DO TOO MUCH, TOO FAST, OR TOO VIGOROUSLY. Listen to your body. We repeat: Releasing an over-abundance of toxic debris all at once will possibly bring on a variety of discomforts even while rebounding aerobics is making you healthier by cleansing the body cells. We want to have you avoid such a reaction, since it may discourage you from continuing with the otherwise excellent movements of this aerobic exercise.

Rebound movements can be classified into four types: basic, intermediate, advanced, and therapeutic. The basic movements are dedicated merely to having you feel comfortable with your timing and balance while standing on the rebound unit. Once you sense your control, you can move on to the various movements that call for bouncing around. Through all the motions, we suggest you breathe deeply — intentionally taking in more air and discarding the habit of shallow breathing, at least while you're rebounding.

The exercise techniques that follow this chapter are designed to lead you into developing some of your own. The ones we have illustrated and described do not exhaust the variety of possibilities, which are limited only by your own imagination. In the four types of rebounding aerobics, the difference between one exercise category and another is mostly a matter of speed of movement, height of the bounce, duration of exercise periods, and intensity of the action. However, all of them provide you with some cardiovascular training effect, which is the primary goal of this book.

In any exercise program you set up, you must make sure that the rebounder you purchase is sturdy enough and designed for safe usage. While rebounding equipment is available at many sporting goods stores, I would recommend a product called Needak produced by Nedak Manufacturing. This fine product is available with an optional stabilizing bar, which acts as a hand rail, for those concerned with keeping their balance. For more information regarding this rebounder, you may write to: Nedak Manufacturing, P.O. Box 776, O'Neill, Nebraska 68763, or you can call them at 1-800-232-5762 or 1-402-336-4083. They also sell other books on rebounding as well as videos.

The Rebounding Techniques

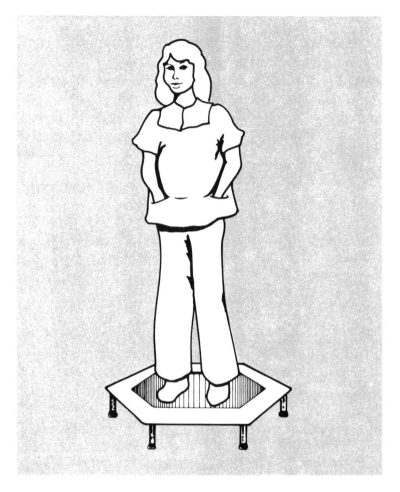

Exercise 1. **Basic.** The "health bounce." Step onto your rebound unit, standing with your feet held apart slightly. Feel your balance. By flexing your ankles begin a small vertical movement up and down. Remain on the mat and increase the height of your bounce a little. Don't lift the soles of your feet, but keep up this bounce for a minute or so just to get used to the movement of rebounding. If necessary, place the rebounding device near a firmly planted object such as a wall or a sturdy piece of furniture and steady yourself on this object as you bounce.

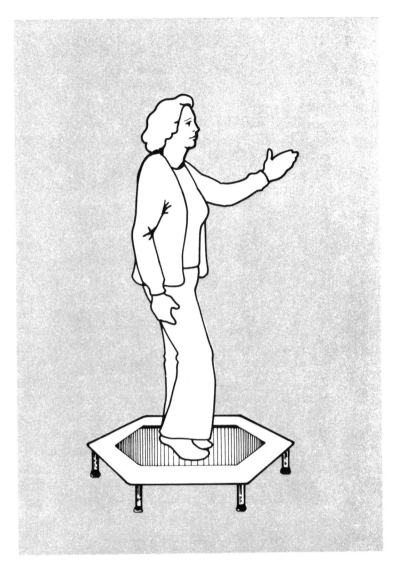

Exercise 2. **Basic.** Alternate the movement of each leg by lifting one heel while your toes remain touching the mat. As you gently thrust the heel into the mat, raise your other heel. Swing your arms as if you're walking in stride. This walking motion is a fine way to warm up and cool down before starting or stopping more vigorous exercise activity.

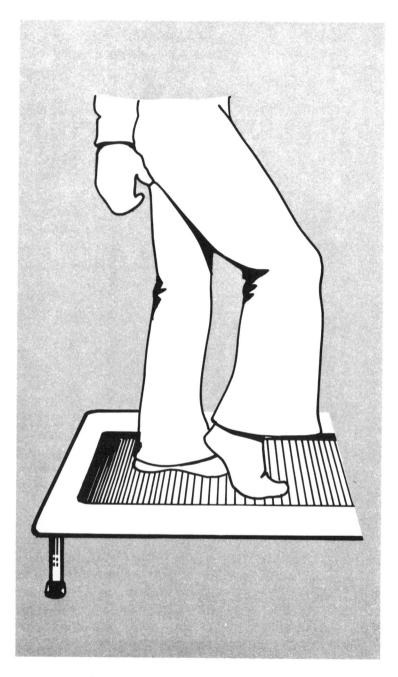

Exercise 2. (cont.)

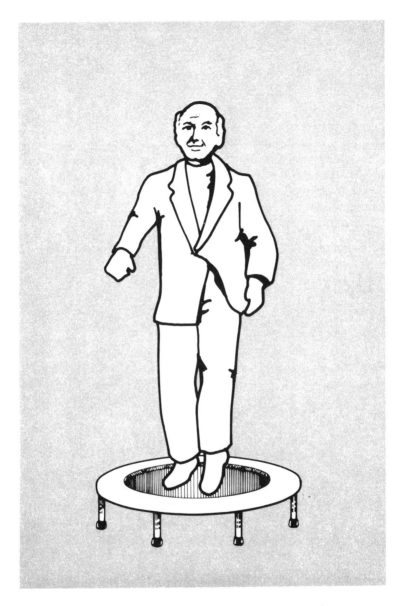

Exercise 3. **Basic.** Begin a very slow jog (known as "slogging") where the feet leave the mat one at a time for an inch or two. Keep checking your balance to make sure you're comfortable with your control. Hold onto an immovable object if required.

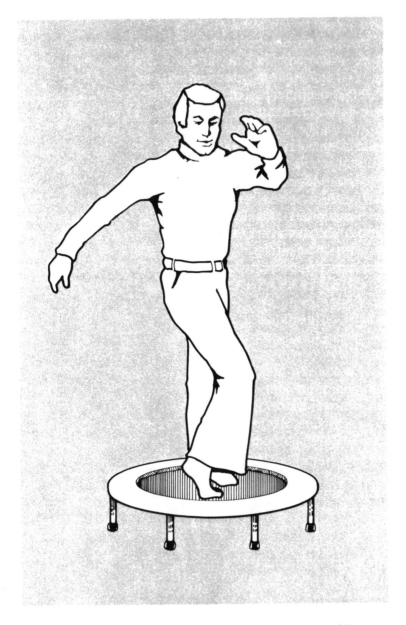

Exercise 4. **Intermediate.** As you progress with your slogging, add a gentle side to side twist with your feet together as you come up on each gentle bounce. This is a good stretching motion for the waist.

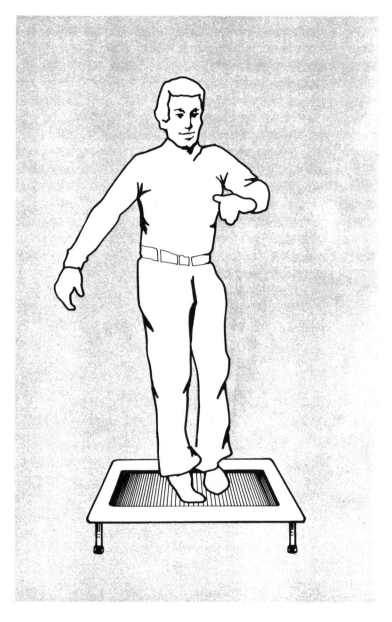

Exercise 4. (cont.)

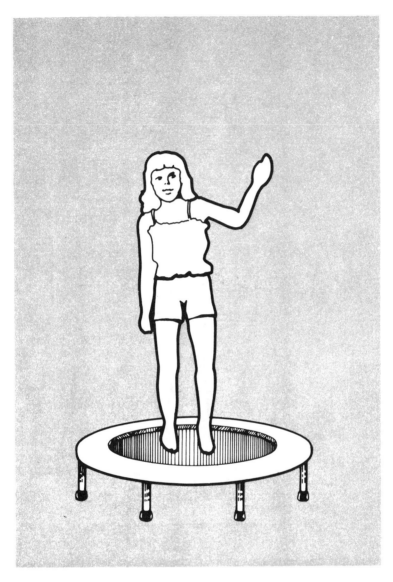

Exercise 5. **Intermediate.** Do an easy vertical bounce with the legs held straight. Rise about three inches above the mat with each bounce so that the force of gravity (G-force) is increased somewhat upon all the cells of the body. You'll be activating your lymphatic system by using this technique.

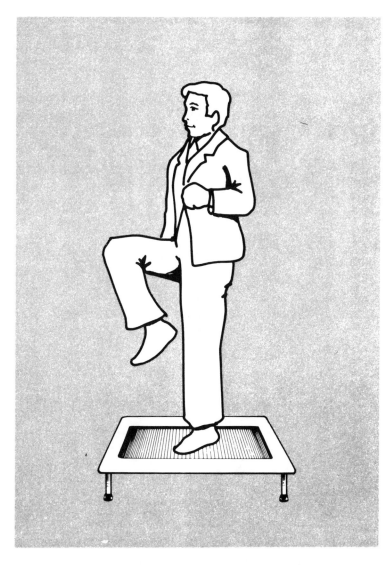

Exercise 6. **Intermediate.** As you are able, progress into a faster jog and then gradually into a run. Lift the legs higher with each step and work up to the point of breathlessness, a condition we call "instant aerobics." Then, cool down to allow your pulse to drop almost to normal, and repeat the whole procedure to develop your cardiovascular efficiency.

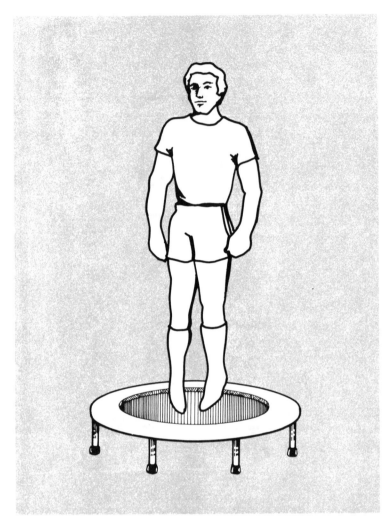

Exercise 7. **Advanced.** Perform a really high vertical bounce of six inches or more to increase the force on your body to 2 Gs or greater. This is a lymphatic exercise dramatic in its effect and is recommended only for a person who is in good condition to withstand the cleansing of possible trapped plasma proteins. This exercise is called the "strength bounce" and it should be built up over a period of time by doing less vigorous rebound exercising first.

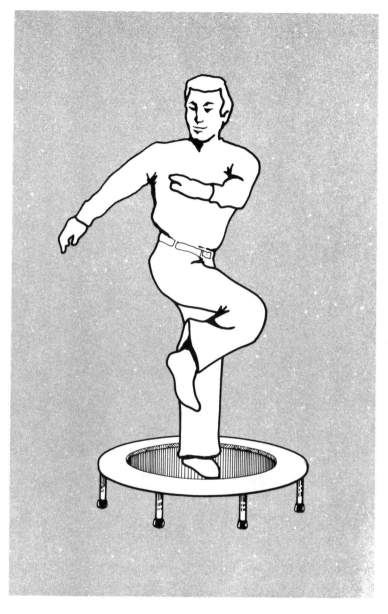

Exercise 8. **Advanced.** Back muscles in good tone are needed to do the side to side twist. Accomplish it by raising the knees higher as you turn each knee inward during the bounce.

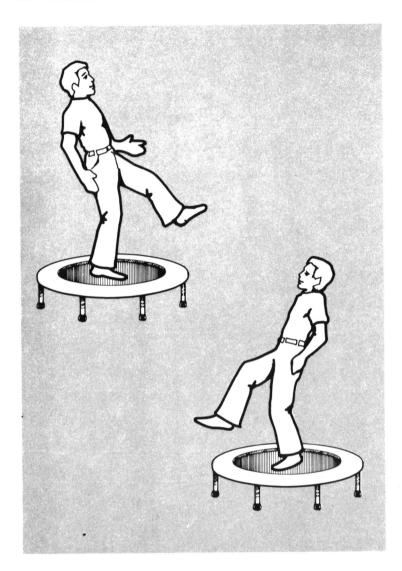

Exercise 9. **Advanced.** The forward kick progresses from mild to vigorous as you swing your arms for balance. It's a lifting of the legs that looks like the soldier's goose step. You may find it advantageous to hold your arms out to the sides for better balance. When your coordination allows, reverse this step to a low to higher back kick.

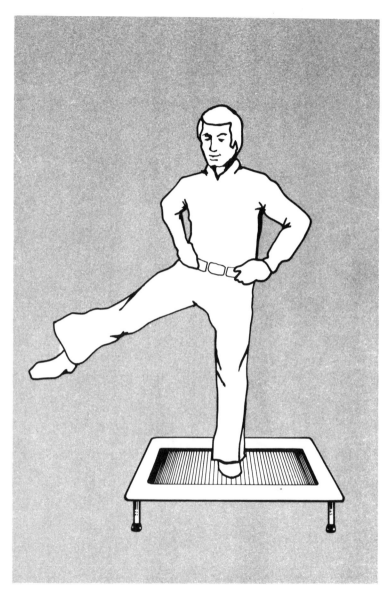

Exercise 10. **Advanced.** The side kick is done by alternating each leg out to the side, low at first and then
stretching higher as you are able. You may prefer to
place your hands on your hips or stretch your arms overhead as you kick from side to side.

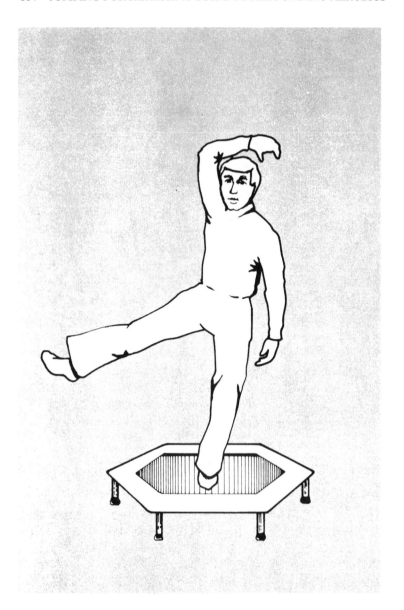

Exercise 10. (cont.)

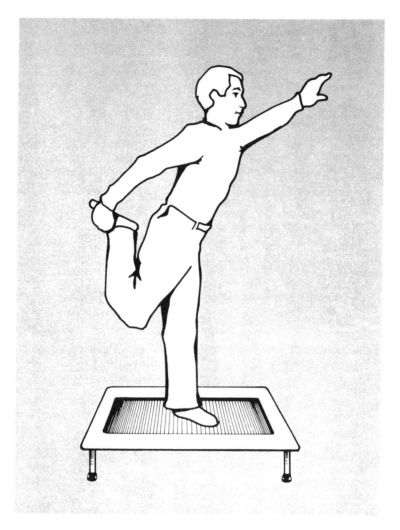

Exercise 11. **Advanced.** For variety's sake, perform balancing exercises such as bouncing on one leg at a time with your hands on hips or your arms outstretched for balance. Try turning a complete circle while on one leg. Hold one foot in back of you while rebounding on the other. Try closing your eyes while doing a few of the basic movements. Practice lower to higher jumping jacks. Of course, you can make up your own combination of exercise variations.

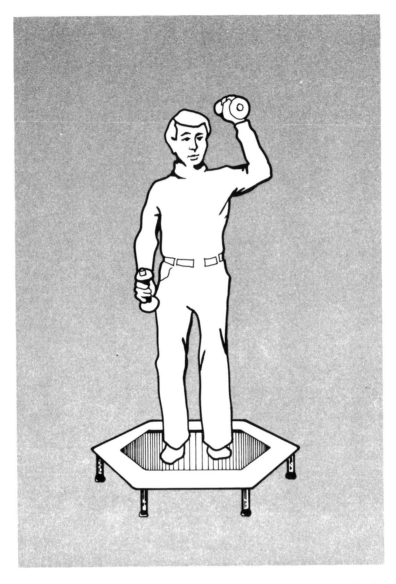

Exercise 12. **Advanced.** To increase your upper body strength (in addition to the G-force strength bounce of exercise 7), add weight by holding light dumbbells or a thick book while bouncing vertically. Gradually increase the weight you hold to increase your strength. You may wish to add weight to your ankles, as well.

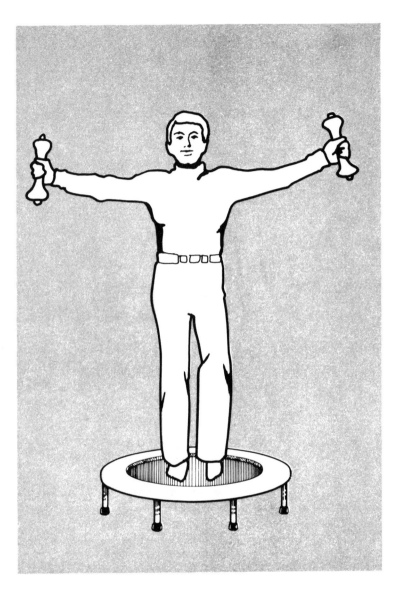

Exercise 12. (cont.)

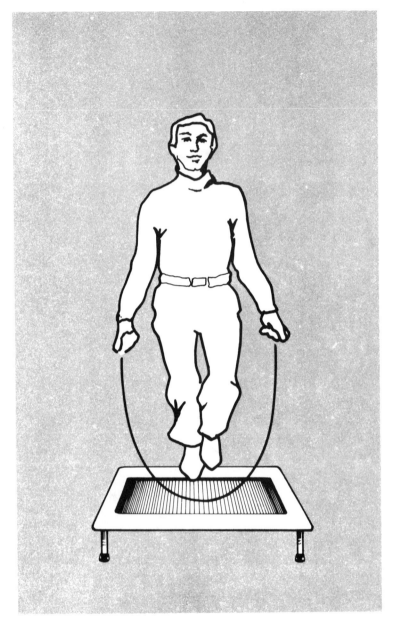

Exercise 13. **Advanced.** Add the fun of skipping rope while rebounding. It enhances your eye-arm-leg coordination.

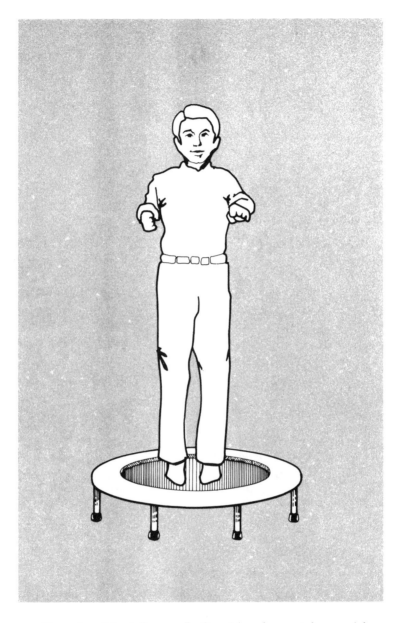

Exercise 14. **Advanced.** Combine isometrics and isotonics to a mild vertical bounce by tightening various muscles when doing some combination stretching movements.

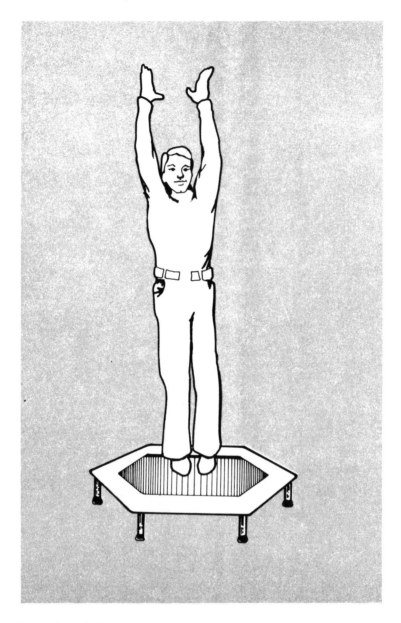

Exercise 14. (cont.)

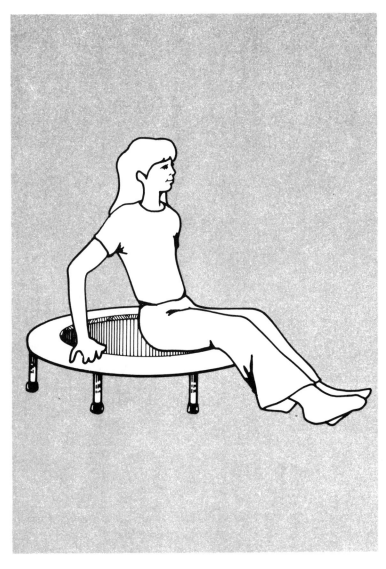

Exercise 15. **Basic.** Sit in the center of the mat with your feet on the floor, place your hands on the rim of the rebound unit, and push your body up and down.

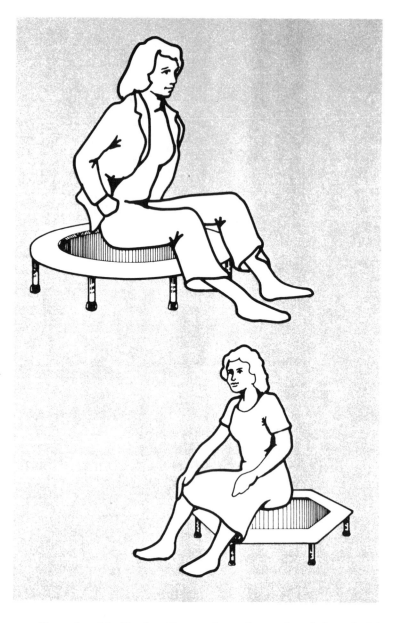

Exercise 16. **Basic.** Sit on the rebound unit but hold your hands off the unit. Then activate a vertical motion by a gentle push with your feet or the vibrating motion of your swinging arms.

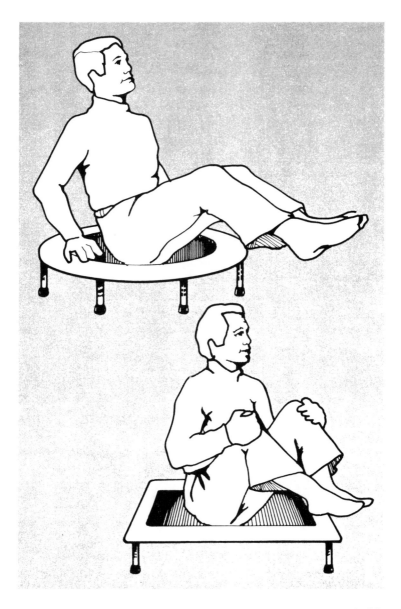

Exercise 17. **Intermediate.** Sit on the mat and lift your feet off the floor. Use your hands for support on the rim if necessary to start your gentle bounce. Then pull your feet onto the rim building on the arm action to activate the motion.

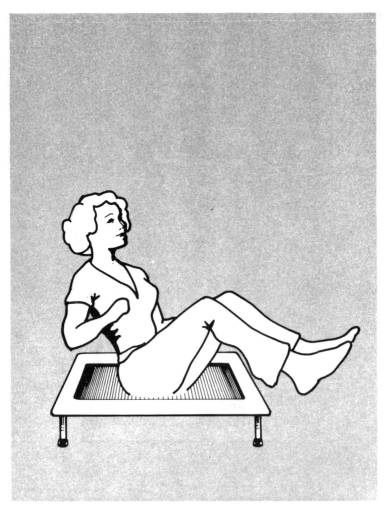

Exercise 18. **Advanced.** While sitting on the mat hold your feet and hands free in the air. Use an up-and-down hip and arm motion to get your body vibrating on the rebound device.

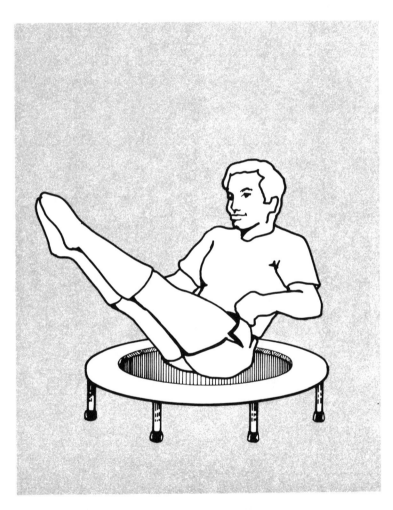

Exercise 19. **Advanced.** For a real "tummy tightener" exercise, form a "V" with your buttocks on the mat and your body and legs bending at a 45-degree angle. Move your body in a pumping motion on the mat by short up-and-down jabs with your arms.

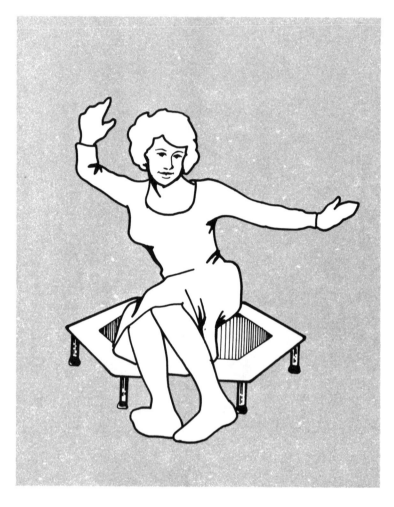

Exercise 20. **Advanced.** Sitting on the mat, do the sitting twist as you swing your arms from side to side while bouncing on one buttock and then the other. This will make you "huff and puff" in a short time. It's an excellent cardiovascular exercise.

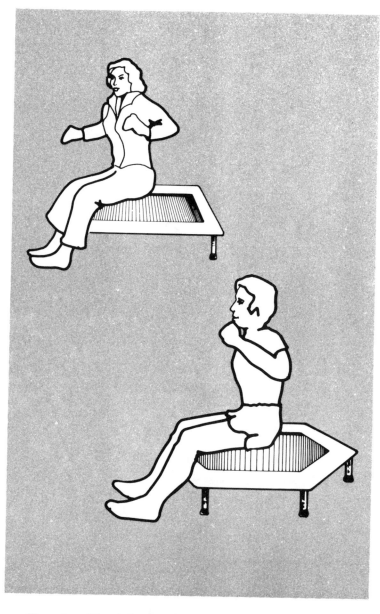

Exercise 21. **Advanced.** When you are in really fit physical condition, sit on the mat and merely perform the high bounce by pumping your arms up and down vigorously.

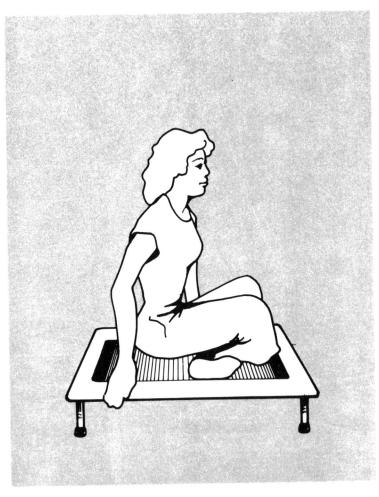

Exercise 22. **Advanced.** Sit cross-legged on the mat with your back straight and do a gentle bounce. Then, with a little push from your feet and a lift with your arms, raise your body a few inches as you rebound up and down for several minutes.

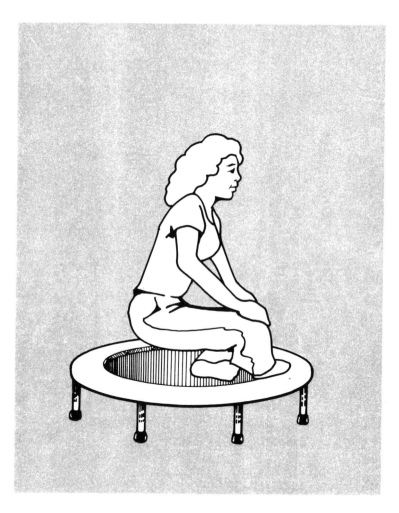

Exercise 22. (cont.)

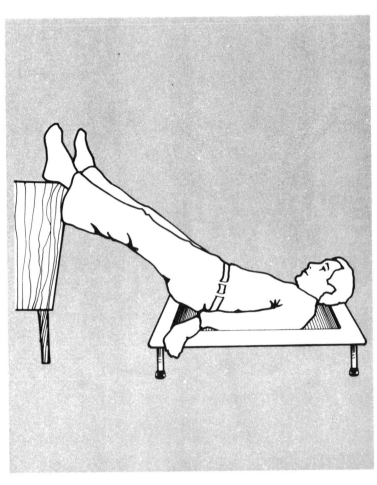

Exercise 23. **Intermediate.** For the purpose of add-ing variety to your techniques, do some rebounding lying down. With your body on the mat (using a small pillow for your head on the rim), prop your feet on a chair, against the wall, or on a couch and gently raise your buttocks in a repeated bounce.

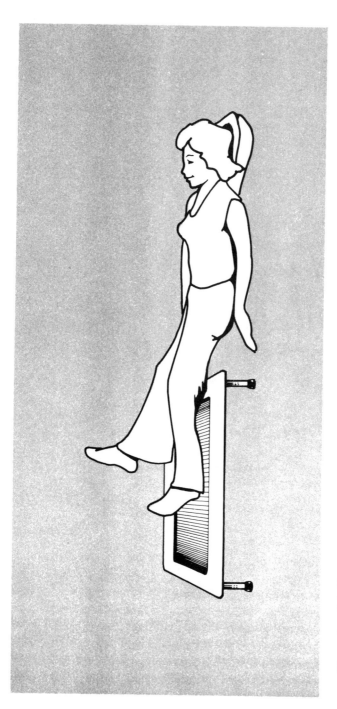

Exercise 24. **Intermediate.** As a good leg relaxation procedure, lie on the floor with your feet on the center of the mat. Begin kicking your feet in a flutter as in swimming the backstroke. Do the flutter kick slowly at first and then increase the tempo.

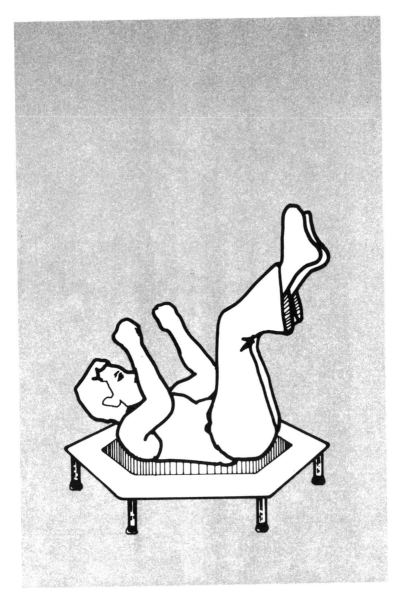

Exercise 25. **Advanced.** Do exercise 23 but hold your legs in the air instead of resting on a piece of furniture. It becomes a real challenge to supply the vertical bounce merely from pumping your arms. This is quite an advanced technique.

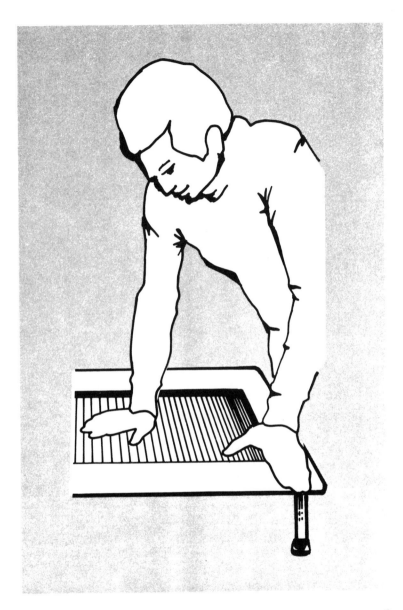

Exercise 26. **Basic.** Place one hand in the center of the mat and press into it for a rapid action of up and down. Next, just use your finger tips for the vibratory effect. Repeat with the other hand. You may find this exercise an aide in overcoming joint stiffness.

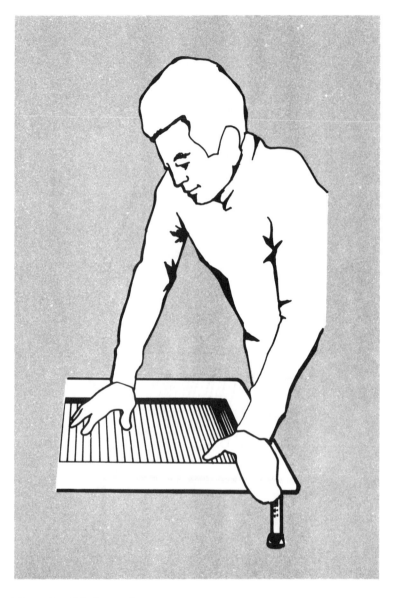

Exercise 26. (cont.)

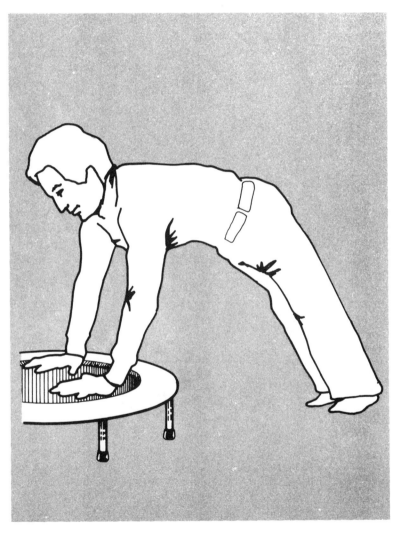

Exercise 27. **Intermediate.** Try doing rhythmical push ups with your hands placed in the center of the mat. This technique strengthens your upper body.

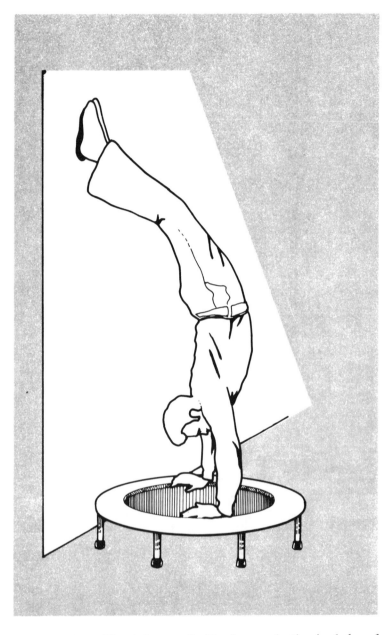

Exercise 28. **Advanced.** Perform rhythmical hand stands on the mat's center. Perhaps you'll need to support your feet against a wall.

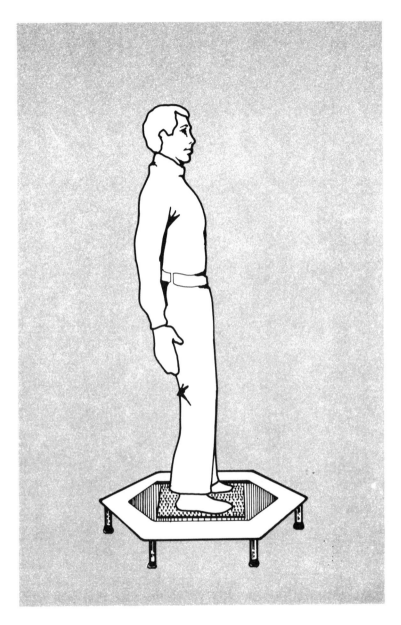

Exercise 29. **Advanced.** Place a knobby door mat or rubber foot massage pad on the mat and go into your gentle bounce. This will stimulate the feet as you get the rebounding effect.

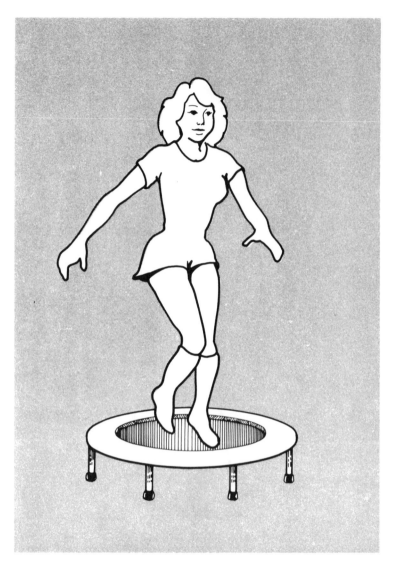

Exercise 30. **Advanced.** With the various illustrated ideas we've supplied, stir your own imagination into action. Put your favorite music on the phonograph, let go of your inhibitions, jump on the mat and go into a dance. Enjoy the fun and excitement of combining your personally designed rebounding routines. Have a good time as you become healthier.

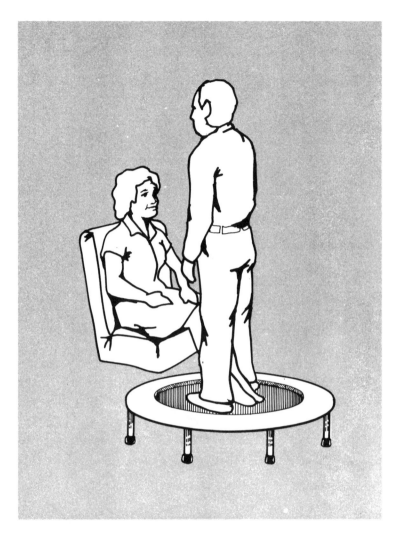

Exercise 31. **Therapeutic.** Certain exercises done for
or by handicapped people are therapeutic in their effect in that they provide muscle action and circulatory
stimulation. The handicapped individual engages in
passive exercise by a second person supplying the rebounding power. Here, the passive person sits on a
chair, in a wheelchair, or on the side of a bed with just
his feet on the mat as the second active person goes into
the gentle bounce.

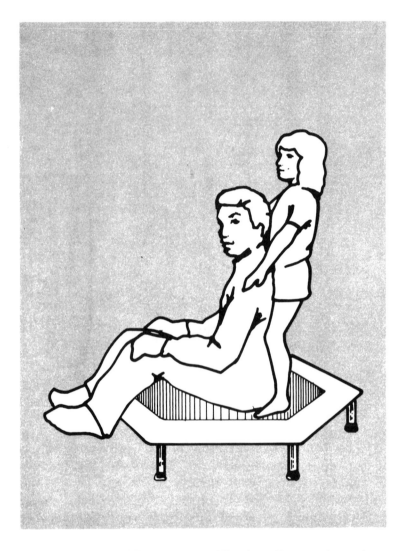

Exercise 32. **Therapeutic.** The handicapped receiver may sit on the rebound mat while resting his or her back against the legs of the active assistant.

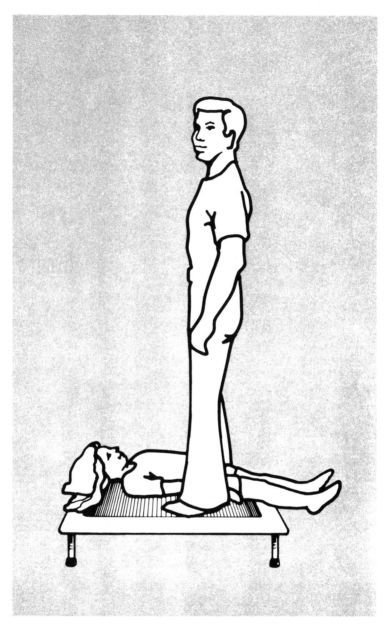

Exercise 33. **Therapeutic.** The handicapped receiver may lay on the mat while the active assistant straddles his or her body and rebounds.

11
The Jarring News About Jogging

In its 205th year the United States is suffering middle-age spread. Its people are more than a billion pounds overweight. This is not surprising considering the calorie content of their favorite drugs, cola drinks, flavored soda pop, alcoholic beverages, and coffee with cream. Last year Americans swallowed 10 billion barrels of sweetened beverages, 621 million gallons of wine and distilled spirits, the equivalent of 49 billion 12-ounce bottles of beer, and an estimated one trillion cups of creamed coffee. With all that sloshing through its system, the populace has to put on pounds.

To offset the intake of calories present in those liquid drugs that we drink, health authorities recommend two types of exercise: One involves vigorously pushing away from the dinner table. The other serves a variety of purposes such as building muscle strength and tone, relieving tension, enhancing skills, improving flexibility, producing weight loss and weight maintenance, and improving the body's general physiological condition, especially the ease with which the heart can supply oxygen to body tissues.

Certain exercises may serve some of these functions well but not others. For example, archery, golf, and bowling when practiced regularly may make you more skillful at the game, but they rarely involve enough continuous activity to condition one's cardiovascular system.

Weight lifting, water-skiing, arm-wrestling, and other isometric exercises may promote strong muscles but are poor cardiovascular conditioners. And nowadays the new craze, perhaps permanently installed as part of American culture, is aerobics to stimulate the lungs to breathe deeply, the heart to pump strongly, and for the cells to give up their wastes effectively. People are engaging in aerobic exercise in order to feel better, look more attractive, lose weight, live longer, and be part of the mainstream of modern life. The chief exercise they've chosen as their aerobic activity is jogging. Many have not yet discovered rebounding aerobics. But they will soon, no doubt, if we have our way.

Yes, America is now on the run. Thousands — maybe millions — have turned to jogging as the alternative to traditional games and sports. Jogging requires the use of lots of oxygen over a relatively long period so that the circulatory system gets conditioned into shape. The main difference between jogging and running is speed. Putting one leg in front of the other at a rate of a mile in seven minutes is running. Taking longer than seven minutes to go a mile is jogging. Some people move at a pace called "slogging" — a very slow jog.

All aerobic exponents — sloggers, joggers, rebound enthusiasts and runners — are all after one thing — cardiovascular fitness. The question is do the benefits of their activity outweigh the risks? Are there dangers connected with jogging? Is rebounding safer and less hard on the body?

Doctors Who Oppose Jogging

Besides the cardiovascular system, another important body structure is the skeletal system. It takes in all the bony parts of the body. If a person ruins his or her ankles, knees, hips and back or other parts of the skeletal system by jogging on a hard surface to enhance the cardiovascular system, what has been the gain? Dr. Gordon Falknor, a Chicago podiatrist, told members attending a meeting of the Illinois Podiatry Association that he has discovered an ailment he calls "jogger's ankle."

"The symptoms are similar to trauma and tendonitis of the achilles tendon just above its attachment to the heel bone," Dr. Falknor explained. He added that tissues of the feet and ankles take a terrific pounding from jogging on concrete or blacktop surfaces. This leads to the eventual breakdown of those tissues.

J.E. Schmidt, M.D., a member of the American Medical Association, who is in private medical practice, suggests that "jogging can kill you." He says it is one of the most wasteful and hazardous forms of exercise which takes more from the body than it gives back. Among the bodily structures most likely to be damaged by jogging are: (1) the sacroiliac joints, (2) the vertebral joints, (3) the veins of the legs, (4) the uterus, (5) the breasts, (6) the abdominal rings (in men), and (7) the heart.

Dr. Schmidt points out that the sacroiliac joint is the "soft underbelly" for the jogging assault. Even without undue violence as that inflicted by jogging or weight lifting, the sacrum frequently tends to sag. It loosens its linkage with the hipbones, causing sacroiliac pains. But add the ballistic impact of jogging to this damaging pressure on top of the sacrum, and you get a sledge hammer jolt like splitting a log, only it will be the lower end of the spine of the jogger that gets jolted each time his foot hits the ground.

The joints of the spine or intervertebral disks are

another jogger-vulnerable body structure, says the medical doctor. Intervertebral disks provide protection from damage by impact. In ordinary functioning, as in walking, the body weight compresses adjacent vertebrae with each step. Under excessive pressure caused by jogging, the outer wall of the disk sometimes bursts and the contents are expelled. The resulting condition — a herniated disk — is known popularly as a slipped disk. It's a jarring experience and really bad news for your back.

The veins of the legs support a column of blood of considerable height. It is not surprising, therefore, that dilated or varicose veins do occur. With jogging, cautions the physician, every thump of the foot makes the blood column pound against the leg veins like a battering ram.

Dr. Schmidt also warned women about jogging dangers to the uterus. This rather loosely fixed organ is situated in the lower part of the pelvis, between the rectum and the bladder. It sprawls over the top of the bladder — carried like a rucksack. Because of the compactness and weight of the uterus, jogging militates in favor of abnormal displacement and other symptoms, said Dr. Schmidt.

He also alerted women to potential damage to their breasts. Female breasts contain no muscles or ligaments in the usual sense. A network of slender fibers provides a tenuous support. These fibers course through the fat, which gives breasts their plump, rounded form, and are attached to the skin. The breasts acquire substantial movement in jogging, and these fibers easily snap. The breasts tend to flatten and droop like deflated balloons, Dr. Schmidt says.

He has just as bad news for men! Abdominal rings in the male are two thinned regions in the lower part of the abdomen. Under pressure, they may permit a part of the intestine through. Even under normal circumstances the abdominal contents may push through an opening, thus causing a hernia.

Dr. Schmidt doesn't even think that jogging is good for the cardiovascular system, especially the heart. He mentions that the heart, a massive organ considering its weight, is not well anchored. It is held in place by little more than connecting arteries. In jogging, every pavement thump is a jar that severely tugs on the major blood vessels.

Finally, Dr. J.E. Schmidt opposes jogging because of other organ casualties. Among the others are the "dropped" stomach, the loose spleen, the floating kidney, and fallen arches.

Jogging Is Not For Everyone

Some people who have been getting up at five o'clock every morning to jog around the block may be in for a rude awakening. Jogging is not for everyone. People with big bones, for example, rarely seem to enjoy jogging because of the extra weight they carry around. But big-boned people do enjoy rebounding because of all its many benefits we've described in prior chapters.

Bernard L. Gladieux, Jr., editor of *The Jogger,* the monthly newsletter of the National Jogging Association, says, "If you are over thirty, you should check with your doctor before you begin any exercise program. If you're over forty, take a treadmill stress test to make sure you're in shape."

Gladieux admitted that joggers can face several physical problems including pulled muscles, nerve irritation and shin splints, the tearing or stretching of tendons in the lower leg. Shin splints produce pain! Nothing like that happens to the rebounder.

If you decide to continue jogging, you can lessen your chance of trouble by doing a series of rebounding exercises accompanied by long, slow stretches before and after the outdoor run. "Not bending and touching your toes five times," cautioned Gladieux. "That type of rapid exercise can cause muscles to bunch up."

"The most insidious problem of all," he continued, "is the overuse syndrome." It strikes people who run too long, too fast and too often and occurs because the body tissues do not get enough rest. If you start suffering, consider changing your schedule. "Someone who runs seven miles every day might be better off running fifteen miles every other day," Gladieux said.

Since joggers are likely to engage in their pastime, we offer some advice. Remember: The pace at which you jog should not leave you collapsing for want of breath. One of the best ways to tell if you are overdoing it is to take the "talk test." If you cannot carry on a conversation while jogging, you are working too hard.

Furthermore, jogging or any other strenuous physical activity can be dangerous to people who are not in good physical condition, especially people with already damaged hearts and fat-clogged arteries. Many men over the age of thirty-five populating industrialized western countries have "hidden" coronary artery disease, and a sudden spurt of running could throw their heart's rhythm out of whack, precipitating a heart attack.

Others for whom strenuous jogging could be dangerous include people with untreated high blood pressure, congestive heart failure, uncontrolled diabetes, skeletomuscular diseases, and obesity. But these health problems are infrequently contraindications for rebounding, since you can adjust your bounce to the movement that has you comfortable. However, we suggest that you should check with your physician before rebounding or doing any other form of exercise, especially jogging.

Ask Yourself These Questions Before Jogging

According to Lenore R. Zohman, the exercise speccialist at Montefiore Hospital and Medical Center in New York City, if you have found the enthusiasm to begin an active jogging program, the quickest way to cool your resolve is to do too much too fast. She said, "Although the muscle aches and twinges of joint pain will pass with perseverance in the program, one serious heart episode is sufficient to dampen the enthusiasm of a whole neighborhood! Exercise can be dangerous to certain people."

Before engaging in an active jogging program, Dr. Zohman suggests you ask yourself a series of pertinent health questions. If you answer "yes" to any of these questions, again we recommend that you consult your physician before beginning to exercise:

1. Has a physician ever said you had heart trouble?

2. Have you ever been the victim of rheumatic fever, growing pains, twitching of the limbs called "St. Vitus Dance," or rheumatic heart disease?

3. Did you ever have, or do you now have a heart murmur?

4. Have you ever experienced a real or suspected coronary occlusion, myocardial infarction, coronary attack, coronary insufficiency, heart attack, or coronary thrombosis?

5. Do you suffer with angina pectoris?

6. Have you ever had an abnormal electrocardiogram taken while you were exercising (such as climbing up and down steps) which was not normal?

7. Have you ever felt pain or pressure or a squeezing sensation in the chest which came on during exercise or walking or any other physical or sexual activity?

8. If you climb a few flights of stairs fairly rapidly, do you experience tightness or pressing pain in your chest?

9. Do you get pressure or pain or tightness in the chest if you walk in the cold wind or get a cold blast of air?

10. Have you undergone bouts of rapid heart action, irregular heart action or palpitations?

11. Have you ever taken digitalis, quinidine or any drug for your heart?

12. Have you ever been prescribed nitroglycerin, sometimes labeled TNG or NTG, or any tablets for chest

pain which you use by placing them under the tongue?

13. Do you have diabetes, high blood sugar, or sugar in the urine now? — At any time in the past?

14. Have you ever or do you now suffer from high blood pressure or hypertension?

15. Have you been on a diet or taken medications to lower your blood cholesterol?

16. Are you more than twenty pounds heavier than you should be?

17. Has there been more than one heart attack or coronary attack or person with heart trouble in your family before age sixty (blood relative)?

18. Do you now smoke more than one pack of cigarettes per day?

19. Are you the victim of any chronic illness?

20. Do you have asthma, emphysema, or another lung condition?

21. Do you get very short of breath on activities which don't make other people similarly short of breath?

22. Have you ever gotten or do you now get cramps in your legs if you walk several blocks?

23. Do you suffer with arthritis, rheumatism, gout or gouty arthritis or a predisposition to gout? Has the uric acid in your blood been found to be high?

24. Do you have any condition limiting the motion of your muscles, joints or any part of the body which could be aggravated by jogging?

Jogging Actually Has Some Value

For the millions of Americans who already have or eventually will succumb to the admonitions to get moving for the sake of their bodies and souls, the prevailing mythology has prompted confusion, anxiety, and inappropriate decisions as to when and how to move. In fact, the list of myths and mistruths about jogging could go on and on, as indicated by what you've just read. There are at least as many myths as there are miles in a marathoner's diary. You might say, when it comes to jogging, "a myth is as good as a mile."

In truth, jogging actually has some value as a builder of fitness even though it gives pain. It is democratic, less expensive, and a quick way to obtain cardiovascular health. Is it for you? Only a number of weeks and months of jogging exploration can begin to answer that question. Obviously, from observing the recent jogging explosion, the answer is "yes" for many.

Jogging is popular because it requires nothing more than a good pair of running shoes, a front door to walk out of, and a willing spirit. It is an effective way to train the cardiovascular system because it uses the largest muscles in the body, the leg muscles. They demand huge quantities of blood and oxygen. This demand is what requires the heart to work harder than usual. And the heart, like any muscle, becomes stronger, more efficient, and more resilient when trained correctly.

Yet, there's an even better way to get the cardiovascular effect you're after. Performing it, you won't get mugged or be bitten by dogs or get rained on or be abused by children or get run down by automobiles or be roasted in the summer and frozen in the winter, or get in the way of another dozen possible discomforts connected with jogging. The better exercise is rebounding regularly.

Rebounding aerobics provides a superior training effect in a shorter period of time. It has none of the dangers of jogging on hard, unyielding surfaces. Rebounding's surface is resilient, cushiony, and comfortable. It's the most efficient, effective, and life preserving exercise as yet developed by mankind. While you're rebounding, you stay relaxed, look great, feel freedom of movement, and have a sense of well-being that you'll not find present in any other aerobic exercise.

Moreoever, this rhythmic endurance exercise of rebounding affords you bionic fitness, something not available from the majority of sports activities and recreational physical movements.

Bionic fitness implies the vitality of a healthy individual who is free from disease or disability. *Bio* means *life* and *onic* refers to the method of putting forth energy — to make vigorous — to energize the human body.

From mechanization and technology, our lives today lend themselves to prolonged periods of inactivity. But bionic fitness offers a program of movement that is not complicated, non-strenuous, and readily available to everyone. Bionic fitness is achieved through rhythmic endurance exercises that cause no muscle soreness. It would be self-defeating to participate in an activity like jogging that leaves you so sore you wouldn't be able to exercise for the next several days. Rhythmic endurance activity encourages you to start your exercise program gradually. Aching muscles are avoided.

The program of rebounding aerobics that we recommend in this book is a rhythmic endurance exercise. It lets you extend your exercise activities to the physical limit best for you. Your endurance and muscle strength increase gradually until you attain bionic fitness.

Other rhythmic endurance exercises include walking, swimming, and running. They encourage stretching and are helpful for improving your muscle tone, respiratory function, blood circulation and general sense of well-being. But these activities are primarily for outdoor use. Rebounding is an easy indoor or outdoor activity that affords rhythmic endurance exercise. It keeps you limber and helps you to shape up if you need to. No other exercise duplicates the benefits of rebounding aerobics. Indeed, the news about jogging is jarring to its enthusiasts, while rebounding is joyful.

12

Food Lobbies Block Nutrition Reports from Public

Basic to improving your body and mind is to eat more nutritiously. Poor nutrition and lack of exercise are the two primary causes for the increase in degenerative diseases in the United States. These are well-established truths that most people recognize. Even the bureaucrats that run our government recognize this, finally, and now they are taking an interest in changing the lifestyles of Americans.

More and more the Federal Government has been taking an active role in setting up national food and nutrition guidelines. In February 1977, the staff of the Select Committee on Nutrition and Human Needs of the United States Senate under the chairmanship of George McGovern, former Senator from South Dakota, released the "Dietary Goals for the United States." Seven dietary goals evolved from the investigations of the Senate Select

Committee which were abhorrent to the food processing industry. They were:

1. To avoid overweight, consume only as much energy (calories) as is expended; if overweight, decrease energy intake and increase energy expenditure.

2. Increase the consumption of complex carbohydrates and "naturally occurring" sugars from about 28 percent of energy intake to about 48 percent of energy intake.

3. Reduce the consumption of refined and processed sugars by about 45 percent to account for approximately 10 percent of total energy intake.

4. Reduce overall fat consumption from approximately 40 percent to about 30 percent of energy intake.

5. Reduce saturated fat consumption to account for about 10 percent of total energy intake; and balance that with polyunsaturated and mono-unsaturated fats, which should account for about 10 percent of energy intake each.

6. Reduce cholesterol consumption to about 300 mg. a day.

7. Limit the intake of sodium by reducing the intake of salt to about five grams a day.

The food processors were incensed by these dietary recommendations for the enhancement of citizen health because they were surely going to cut into the sales and profits of the processed food business. Consequently, it set into motion the powerful food industry lobby which acted against the advocates of a return to localized agriculture and a simpler, less processed food supply. The lobby, in fact, was powerful enough to have the Select Committee abolished December 31, 1977. Under the Senate reorganization plan, responsibility for any additional dietary investigations fell to the Subcommittee on Agriculture, Nutrition, and Forestry.

Before abolishment, however, Senator McGovern's committee prepared another report, "Guidelines for Food Purchasing in the United States." The "Guidelines" were intended to complement the Select Committee's first report on "Dietary Goals." They were:

1. Avoid premixed, ready-to-eat and refined foods in favor of fresh foods.

2. Base food-buying decisions on taste, price, and nutrition knowledge rather than advertising.

3. As much as possible, purchase foods through co-operatives and farmers markets, or grow your own.

In following the three guidelines, the consumer would not only effectively achieve the Dietary Goals but save a substantial amount of money and also save energy and other resources. Until now, the report has been buried by the new nutrition subcommittee of the Senate Agriculture Committee. In an interview, Marshall Matz, special counsel for that subcommittee, said that he seriously doubts "the possibility of our ever publishing it."

Why doesn't the Government give us the information? Our tax dollars paid for its investigation.

The Guidelines Come into My Hands

Knowing of the work of my fellow medical journalist, Nick Mottern of Millwood, Virginia, we took steps to acquire the "Guidelines" in an indirect way from him. Mr. Mottern is a former staff member of the Senate Select Committee on Nutrition and Human Needs. He was directly responsible for writing the guidelines report, simultaneously with the work on the "Dietary Goals" report, both of which he began in the spring of 1976.

Mottern's guidelines take a firm anti-big-business stance, noting that advertising, processing, packaging, and transportation devour a major portion of the food dollar. The buried report says that consumers have the most control over their diet when preparing meals "from scratch" and that, given current manufacturing and labeling practices, reliance on staple foods is the only means by which the consumer can adequately control consumption of fat, sugar, salt, and additives.

He noted that once-cheap energy had allowed Americans to develop a large, centralized food system that made heavy processing and long-distance transportation the norm, but now that high energy costs are with us we need to do more direct farmer-to-consumer food buying.

Why did Nick Mottern release the unauthorized report without Government sanction? He said, "I felt the climate inside the committee, with many members opposed to or unsympathetic to the dietary goals, was such that the report would never have been published."

Of course, Mr. Mottern is no longer with the committee. He left almost three years ago following a feud over revisions of the dietary goals.

Specific Guidelines in Mottern's Report

As one of the authors of the 1977 "Dietary Goals" and the chief author of the new "Guidelines for Food Purchasing", Mottern said, "People have to begin looking to alternatives. We can't just go on saying conditions aren't good. The rising cost of food is a tremendous problem. We have become such an urban society, so cut off from the food supply, that we feel we have no control over what we put on the table or how it gets there."

The U.S. Government confidential report states that Americans could realize substantial savings on food bills and enhance their own nutrition if they avoided highly processed foods, bought more dried foods in bulk and more fresh foods, and made more purchases through cooperatives and farmers markets.

For the first time published under the copyright laws anywhere, the specific official guidelines are as follows:

1. **In preparing meals, to the degree possible, substitute fresh and processed food staples for pre-mixed, ready-to-eat, refined and/or substitute foods.**

Processed staples include foods processed solely for ιe purpose of preservation, such as canned and frozen ;getables as well as those processed for use as ingred-·nts, such as flour and vegetable oil.

Pre-mixed, refined foods referred to in the report as ighly processed foods and not recommended include:

Soft drinks
Juice substitutes
Sugared fruit drinks
Artificial fruit drinks
Refined breakfast cereals
Breakfast drink mixes and bars
Frozen breakfast entrees
Packaged donuts, buns, cakes, pies
Cake, cookie and other pastry mix
Potato and corn chips and puffs
All candy
Infant formula
Bottled infant complete meals
Seasoned meat extenders and "helpers"
Prepared salad dressings and mayonnaise
Prepared tarts and waffles
Dessert mixes
Prepared doughs
Prepared cheese and other dips
Meat, egg, and dairy substitutes
Coffee creamer substitutes
Luncheon meats
Frozen dinners and entrees
Frozen vegetables in sauces
Canned and packaged soups
Prepared tomato and other sauces

2. **Rely solely on nutrition knowledge, nutrition label-ıg and grading (where available), taste, and price in ıaking food purchasing decisions; avoid making de-isions on the basis of brand name advertising and dvertising aimed at increasing the consumption of a articular commodity.**

3. **Purchase food through consumer cooperatives and lirect farmer to consumer markets, and grow your own ɔod to the degree possible. If consumer cooperatives**

and/or direct markets do not exist in your area, organize them where possible.

Households with Health Problems Change Their Diets

A survey of 1,500 households conducted in 1976 by the U.S. Department of Agriculture found that diet changes were made to contend with health problems or to avoid them. (Table VI from the report shows the numbers of households in which there were health problems and the percentage of those making dietary changes.) The changes made most often were: avoidance of sweets and snacks, fried foods, fatty red meat, ice cream, and soft drinks. The leading additions to diets were lowfat milk and cheese, lean red meat, fish, fresh fruits, fresh vegetables, poultry, and broiled and baked foods. In general, diet-conscious consumers sought to cut down on items relatively high in sugar, saturated fats and oils, and in many cases, calories.

Table VI

HOUSEHOLDS WITH HEALTH PROBLEMS AND THOSE MAKING DIET CHANGES

Health Problem	% Households Having Health Problems	% Households with Health Problems Changing Diet
Overweight	30	64
High Blood Pressure	22	55
Allergy	20	31
Heart Disease	9	62
Kidney Disease	8	40
High Blood Cholesterol	8	88
Diabetes	7	75

Source:
Are Health Concerns Changing the American Diet?
Judith Lea Jones, National Economic Analysis Division,
Economic Research Service, 1976.

Questions arise relating to this U.S. Department of Agriculture study: Why do household members wait until a health problem strikes before they change their nutrition for the better? Why is the Government holding back on release of this information that would improve the health of the nation?

Convenience Foods Cause Disease

Mottern's report condemns the use of convenience foods. He writes: "There is no way for the consumer, under current labeling and processing practices, to systematically determine the nutritional characteristics of commercially prepared foods." Reading the label tells you very little. Furthermore, the time actually saved through the use of highly processed foods is not as substantial as it sometimes seems. The desire for convenience foods is also robbing Americans of a certain amount of the pleasure of eating.

In summary, the U.S. Department of Agriculture report suggests that there are substantial consumer benefits from investing more time in the selection and preparation of food.

New ways of home preparation, such as freezing of foods and involvement of all family members in food purchasing and preparation, can provide at once more home-made convenience and more pleasure.

In a speech entitled "Diet Change and Public Policy," presented at the Conference on Future Directions in Health Care, February 15-16, 1977, in New York City, Beverly Winikoff, M.D., a nutritionist with the Population Council, spoke against commercial advertising of foods that emphasizes the positive without mentioning the negative. She said:

> . . . it is not clear that any food — even the most nutritious or wholesome — should be promoted commercially. In the process of advertising, food items are presented as being in competition with other foods or food groups. The tenor of advertising done by industry associations transmits the message — implicitly or ex-

plicitly — that that group's particular product is necessary to good health. A corollary of such messages is that the more of the product consumed, the better for the health of the consumer. This is rarely, if ever, the case and is an inappropriate emphasis for nutrition information.

Convenience food technology has been criticized for lacking good nutritional quality. In testimony before the Select Committee, September 30, 1977, Dr. Kent K. Stewart, a staff member of the United States Department of Agriculture's Nutrient Composition Laboratory, said "We have little or no data for any nutrients" in fast foods, convenience foods, beverages, institutional food, including restaurant food, and snacks.

Food technology, which concerns itself primarily with the preservation and manipulation of food, has developed as a science faster than the capacity of nutritionists to measure food technology's impact on nutrition. In fact, the main objective of the food technologist is to develop preservation methods and invent new foods and processes so that an expanding variety of products may be marketed in an ever-increasing geographic area. He is not interested in supplying the highest level of nutrition. Instead, the food technologist concerns himself with color, flavor, texture, appearance, and stability of the product. The processed food industry appears to consider nutritionists "persona non grata" and seldom includes them in research and development teams, except perhaps in companies marketing pet food.

The above information is paraphrased from the Government's own secret report. It relates specifically to nutrition and human needs, but the Government has buried this information. The only way we have been able to publish a small part of it here is through the courageous act of the former Senate Staff Member who made the "Guidelines for Food Purchasing in the United States" available indirectly to us. To get it, we had to use our credentials as former president of the Connecticut Chapter of the Natural Food Associates and as medical journalists anxious to educate American taxpayers. After-all our money paid for this report which has been buried.

Benefits from Using the Guidelines

If the American public had full access to the Government's food purchasing guidelines it would gain certain nutritional benefits:

1. **Reliance on staple foods is the only means, given current manufacturing and labeling practices, by which the consumer can adequately control consumption of fat, sugar, salt, and food additives.**

2. **By reducing and/or eliminating refined and fabricated foods from the diet, the consumer can maximize the potential for obtaining important trace elements.**

Note: A fabricated food is one that is constructed, usually with the help of food additives, from factors that have been refined from staple foods. In the book, *Orthomolecular Nutrition* (Keats Publishing, 1978), Abram Hoffer, M.D., Ph.D. and Morton Walker, D.P.M. call fabricated products "food artifacts." They are usually marketed as substitutes for other naturally occurring foods, principally meat and dairy products. For example, texturized vegetable protein, made from refined products of soybeans, is sold as a meat substitute.

A refined food is one from which certain factors have been removed by mechanical or chemical means to make the food more appealing or long-lived. The most widely consumed refined products are those made from white flour, milled white from whole grain wheat. Refining does nothing to enhance the nutritional value of a food; instead, it depletes its health-producing properties.

3. **By overlooking the influence of brand name food advertising, as well as advertising of various food companies, the consumer can develop a more healthful, varied and appealing diet.**

Note: "The Dietary Goals for the United States" says that in 1975, about $1.15 billion was spent on food advertising in this country, and that 70 percent of television advertising time promotes "low-nutrient, generally high-calorie foods," currently. It says that more than 50 percent of television advertising dollars are negatively related to health. TV advertising of processed foods is destructive to life and health owing to the product messages it beams to the American public.

4. **Consumer food co-operatives, direct marketing and gardening offer the opportunity to increase consumption of vegetables and fruit and at the same time increase food knowledge and, in the case of gardens, self-sufficiency.** In the event there is another war of nuclear proportions, the only people who will survive after the initial wounding and dying are those who grow their own food. There won't be any stores, shops, or supermarkets from which to buy it.

Food and Energy Wastes

Wasted energy and wasted nutrients in food are simultaneous Government and industry undertakings. As mentioned already, just three and one-half years ago Senator George McGovern, Chairman of the U.S. Senate Select Committee on Nutrition and Human Needs issued the report, entitled *Dietary Goals for the United States.* "I was pleasantly surprised, if not shocked, by the reception of that report," said Senator McGovern. "I've seen a good many government documents published in the twenty-three years I've been here in Washington. I've never seen one that had a more striking impact than this one. It's been a best seller at the Government Printing Office. It's been widely discussed by members of the Congress, throughout the executive branch, the medical profession, health groups — particularly preventive health groups — so that all around the country and indeed around the world the report is being discussed and circulated as a measurement by which the question of nutrition could be discussed."

The impact of the "Dietary Goals" has been so great on the food processing industry that giant processing companies have consequently taken steps to bury this second report which had been scheduled for publication just one year later. The recommendations of *Guidelines for Food Purchasing in the United States* have never been revealed. The American public doesn't even know of their existence, until now.

Mottern's report additionally ties together food waste and energy waste. Written over a two-year period and based on testimony from nutrition committee hearings, various reports and consultations with nutritionists, food technologists and economists, the report shows how food processing and transportation of the processed products waste tremendous quantities of energy resources in coal, oil, and other sources of power. The waste comes about for purposes of unnecessary food processing, strictly as a means of building industrial profits. Not only does this power expenditure not add anything of a nutritional nature to the final food products, it actually squanders the natural nutrients in the original food.

Food and Energy Are Taken For Granted

Nick Mottern says that his report provides simple guidelines that seem to make sense to people almost intuitively. It helps them to sort their way through a very confusing array of advertising, nutrition advice, dietary advice — the whole business. But it may never be read because it steps on the toes of powerful interests in agribusiness and the Washington representatives who are paid by them.

"Food has been taken so for granted," said Mottern. "I think it's something that people are just catching on to. I think that people don't really understand how basic food is. We are so used to having a plentiful food supply, one that is appealing to most people. There hasn't been any appraisal of food as a fundamental thing — or what changes in eating patterns would mean to people, to energy, and to structure of agribusiness. The whole development of agribusiness hasn't really been studied very much.

"In terms of the average person addressing food in the same way as he or she would address gasoline, for instance, at this point there is a certain uneasiness about food . . . In general, I think that people feel uneasy about things that are given to them, completed for them, to consume," said Mottern. "Maybe some of that food is perfectly safe; but it's the idea that it's estranged from them — the most basic thing of life is estranged from them. When that happens, estrangement in other things is a natural consequence."

Mottern did his Senate Committee investigations and wrote the report to educate the public so that they would have information with which to make changes in the system. Their estrangement must be allayed by giving them the ability to correct a corrupted expenditure of energy for unnecessary food processing. Energy is getting in short supply, as anyone paying $1.25 per gallon for home heating oil knows only too well.

Energy Use in the Food System

Guidelines for Food Purchasing in the United States prepared for the Senate Select Committee on Nutrition and Human Needs but released without authorization of the Senate Committee on Agriculture, Nutrition, and Forestry which absorbed the McGovern Committee in January 1978, says that the food system in the United States accounts for at least 17 percent of the total energy demand for the nation. Also, another report, *Energy Use in the Food System*, published by the Federal Energy Administration, says that the 17 percent estimate is probably too low because there are certain components of the food system which use energy but were not available for calculations.

Fifty-five percent of the energy use in the food system is devoted to functions of processing and distribution. About 8.5 calories of energy are required to produce one calorie of food energy (an exceedingly conservative estimate). The energy expenditure for processing food has been increasing steadily since 1940. An article by John and Carol Steinhart, appearing in *Science,* April 1974, estimates that "to feed the entire world with a U.S.-type food system, almost 80 percent of the world's annual energy expenditure would be required just for the food system."

The Steinharts have calculated that energy use by the food processing industry has tripled over the last thirty years. This increase has paralleled the increased marketing potential of highly processed foods. A United States Department of Agriculture study, *The U.S. Food and Fiber Sector: Energy Use and Outlook,* predicts that by next year the processing industry's share of total food energy use "will increase from 28 percent of the total to 40 percent, as more foods are processed to higher levels of convenience. The greatest increase will be in frozen specialities — TV dinners, pizzas, and other snack foods." This will double the need for British Thermal Units of energy.

For many products, the amount of energy used is greater in processing than in production of the original crop. For example, 200 calories are expended in growing corn, but processing and canning corn require 1,000 calories. Processing frozen potatoes requires more than three-and-a-half times as much energy as for fresh potatoes. In fact, Mottern's report shows the energy use for ten different potato processes:

Table VII

Food Processing	BTU's Per Serving
Frozen Potatoes	7000
Freeze-Dried Potatoes	6000
Refrigerated Potatoes	4000
Canned Potatoes	3800
Microwave-Dried Potatoes	3000
Retort-Pouched Potatoes	2900
Spray-Dried Potatoes	2250
Granule-Dried Potatoes	2200
Flake-Dried Potatoes	2150
Fresh Potatoes	1800

To conserve energy and eat more nutritionally, the "Guidelines" recommend that the consumer increase consumption of fresh food and decrease consumption of highly processed food. Purchase food in bulk when possible to avoid excess packaging. This will result in substantial energy savings as well as the reduced loss in resources used in packaging.

Consume Less Meat We're Advised

The authorized but unpublished report also recommends that the consumer should stop energy waste by eating differently: "eat less meat and leaner meat; less animal fats and oils; less sugary foods and alcoholic beverages. Eat more grain products." The National Livestock and Meat Board really screams in rebuttal, but there is no denying, according to the Steinharts, that energy use in food production in the U.S can be cut by 50 percent over the next 75 years. They suggest a 50 percent reduction in consumption of meat and discontinuation of the use of grain finishing of beef.

In *Science,* November 22, 1975, David Pimentel estimates that it takes five kilograms of vegetable and fish protein as animal feed to produce one kilogram of animal protein for human consumption. Consequently, although vegetable protein is not as complete a protein as animal protein, greater use of vegetable protein can save resources in terms of land, fertilizer, pesticides, and petroleum.

Plant protein requires two to thirteen pounds of fertilizer compared to eight to 148 pounds for an equivalent amount of animal protein. Gerald Leach said in *Energy and Food Production,* published in 1976:

> The question is not whether animal products are a wicked luxury, but when is enough? The farm outputs and dietary intakes of animal products have been rising steadily over the past 20 years ... Quite a reversal of this trend could save a substantial amount of fossil fuel energy and release a lot of land for a less intensive and less resource profligate type of farming.

Grain production — oats, corn, soybeans and wheat — consumes the least amount of energy. Apples, grapes, pears, peaches and sugar beets are in the intermediate range of energy intensity. Green beans, lettuce, broccoli, tomatoes, celery and cauliflower are in high ranges of energy intensity, largely because more fertilizer, pesticides and irrigation are used in current methods of production.

Two of the most energy intensive food processes are beet sugar refining and corn milling, especially when they are processed into confectionery products. Dark rye flour and whole wheat flour provide the highest nutritional value for energy consumed, and chocolate bars, granulated sugar and shortening provide the least.

Grow Food in a Home Garden

The "Guidelines" suggest that we eat only enough food to meet our personal energy needs. Obesity is an energy as well as a health problem. If all those people who are overweight in this country went on appropriate diets, the energy savings during the dieting period would be equivalent to 1.3 billion gallons of gasoline.

The savings every year thereafter as the population maintained ideal weight would be equivalent to three-quarters of a billion gallons of gasoline a year. About 900,000 average U.S. autos getting fourteen miles per gallon, traveling 12,000 miles a year could be fueled annually with this savings. Also, this annual energy savings would more than supply the electrical demands of Boston, Chicago, San Francisco, and Washington, combined each year.

Body energy could be expended for healthy weight maintenance if people would grow more food in their gardens at home. The average energy savings of growing vegetables at home averages 45 percent. Energy can further be increased if the garden is hand-spaded, if organic rather than chemical fertilizer is used as well as biological rather than chemical pesticides.

Purchase Food Directly from Farmers

The buried Government report says that food co-operatives are less energy wasting than the current retail food distribution system. Cooperative buying clubs save energy since purchasing is done by a few individuals for the many, thus saving the gasoline individual consumers would expend on trips to supermarkets.

"More directly," says the report, "cooperatives can assist in reducing energy consumption by acting as purchasing agents which can stimulate more localized food production. The energy benefits of more localized production are clear with respect to transportation energy costs."

Chicken broiler production is concentrated in the Southeast and South Central states, far from population centers. Fruit and vegetable production is concentrated in California, Florida, and Texas, across the country from major consumption centers. Between 1963 and 1967 alone, the average length of haul for canned fruits and vegetables increased from 658 miles to 865